ALTITUDE ILLNESS:
Prevention & Treatment

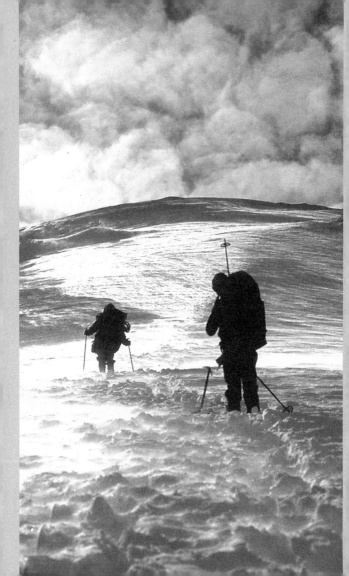

ALTITUDE ILLNESS:
Prevention & Treatment

HOW TO STAY HEALTHY AT ALTITUDE:
FROM RESORT SKIING TO
HIMALAYAN CLIMBING

Stephen Bezruchka, M.D., M.P.H.
SECOND EDITION

THE MOUNTAINEERS BOOKS

THE MOUNTAINEERS BOOKS
*is the nonprofit publishing arm of The Mountaineers Club,
an organization founded in 1906 and dedicated to the
exploration, preservation, and enjoyment of outdoor
and wilderness areas.*

1001 SW Klickitat Way, Suite 201, Seattle, WA 98134

© 2005 by The Mountaineers Books

First edition 1994. Second edition: first printing 2005, second printing 2009.

Published simultaneously in Great Britain by Cordee,
3a DeMontfort Street, Leicester, England, LE1 7HD

Manufactured in Canada

Project Editor: Laura Drury   Copy Editor: Joeth Zucco
Cover and Book Design: The Mountaineers Books
Layout: Peggy Egerdahl
All photographs by the author unless otherwise noted.

Cover photograph: *The Jungfrau, Switzerland* © Digital Stock
Frontispiece: *Mount Lucania, Icefield Range, Yukon*

Library of Congress Cataloging-in-Publication Data

Bezruchka, Stephen.

  Altitude illness : prevention and treatment : how to stay
healthy at altitude: from resort skiing to Himalayan climbing / by
Stephen Bezruchka.-- 2nd ed.
     p. cm.
  Includes bibliographical references and index.
  ISBN 0-89886-685-5
  1. Mountain sickness. 2. Altitude, Influence of. I. Title.
  RC103.M63B49 2005
  616.9'893--dc22

                                    2005008270

 Printed on recycled paper

To those who died of altitude illness

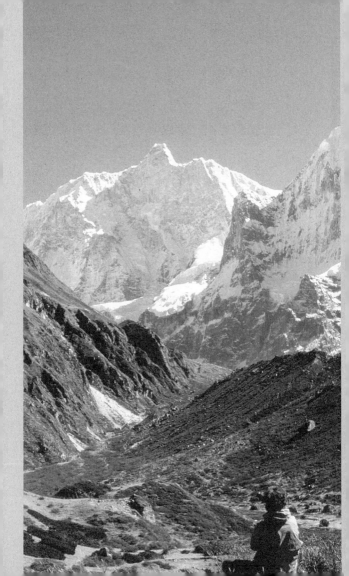

Contents

Jannu from north, Nepal

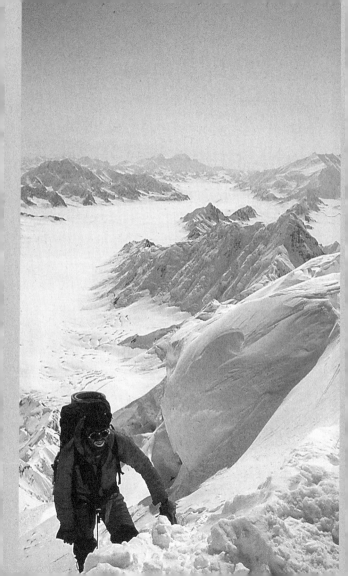

Preface

"I get high with a little help from my friends," sang the Beatles, in the spirit of the '60s. Today more and more people want to get high, and they usually do it with friends, but the way up is by climbing. The euphoria that comes with gaining altitude has been known to the Europeans for centuries. Upon attaining a summit, several of my German friends would say "Und now we enjoy the high altitude." The heights are to be savored, but it is easy to get sick there too.

This portable book is designed to travel to altitude with you. Use it to

- prepare for going to altitude.
- recognize the symptoms of acute mountain sickness.
- assess altitude-related problems accurately.
- decide on treatment methods.
- prevent serious complications.

East Ridge Mount Logan, Yukon

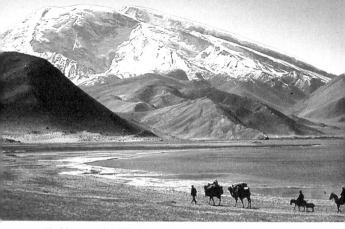

Kirghiz nomads, Little Karakul Lake, Western China

The information presented here is suitable for skiers, climbers, hikers, and trekkers heading to international destinations such as Quito, Ecuador; Lhasa, Tibet; Everest Base Camp; or high altitude sites in the United States, such as Mount McKinley (Denali), Alaska or Mammoth Mountain, California. Whether a novice going to altitude for the first time, a seasoned hiker, or a veteran Himalayan climber, all will find this book an essential piece of gear.

Many of the treatments and medical advice presented in this book are not FDA approved. *Altitude illness* is a nascent area of study that does not allow large, controlled clinical trials for a number of reasons. One obstacle is that altitude illness affects relatively small numbers of people idiosyncratically. Second, high altitude terrain makes research difficult. Third, more and more people with various preexisting health problems are going high. Studying the effect of altitude on other health conditions is not something done well by mainstream medical science, so don't expect more than informed judgment to be presented in this volume. When far from expert help and facilities, use the information presented here to make the best of a difficult situation. Don't consider any drug treatments for altitude illness without first discussing them with a knowledgeable doctor and verifying drug dosages and indications.

This edition presents updates on various treatment modalities, including new drugs that may have some benefit. In the past decade, exposure to "thin air" has become fashionable. People with many preexisting health conditions have successfully ventured to the heights, and guidelines for these conditions are presented. We now have a better idea of who will get sick at altitude. This includes people living at the high terrain you visit. Language and cultural issues increase the difficulties of providing care for them. With the increased numbers up high, there are more cases of people getting sick with conditions other than altitude illness. Considering the causes of ill health at altitude requires increased judgment, something that is difficult to do in the rarefied atmosphere when brains don't function well.

I ponder the role of books providing helpful advice in the new information age. The Internet provides the universe's biggest haystack wherein you may find many needles, some that will sew for you and others that may stab or prick you. For the near future, Wi-Fi access may not be possible on high, and I expect continued need for small volumes such as this where everything you need to know is compactly presented. I am reminded of a colleague who perused the Internet looking for advice for the chest pain symptoms his wife began having. He didn't follow the common-sense protocols widely advertised, and his spouse died while he was surfing.

I have no financial interest in any endeavor related to altitude outside of this book and my other books on Nepal and travel medicine.

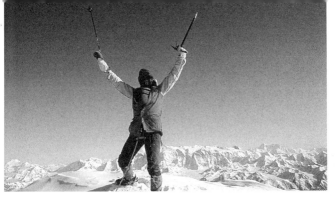

Author on Mount Lucania, Saint Elias Range, Yukon

Acknowledgments

I am grateful to Buddha Basnyat, Peter Hackett, Jim Litch, David Scott, David Shlim, and Eric Swenson for help with this edition. As well I have benefited immensely from communications with users of the first edition and with people concerned about going high with various chronic illnesses. Joeth Zucco deftly edited the manuscript to aid understanding. Thank you all.

How to Use This Book

Before taking a trip up high, read chapters 1, 2, 3, and 7, decide which drugs you might consider carrying, and then discuss them with a knowledgeable doctor. During a trip, if you suspect that you or your companions have altitude illness and need to assess the situation, turn to chapter 4 and follow the steps to diagnose a specific disorder. If you or a companion has a preexisting health condition, read chapter 6 and consider a shakedown trip near home where there are easier options for dealing with problems that may occur. Look over the case studies in chapter 8 as well as questions and answers in chapter 9 that present important material in a way that many people find helpful.

New terms are italicized the first time they are used and are defined in the glossary. Units are given in feet, followed by meters in parentheses.

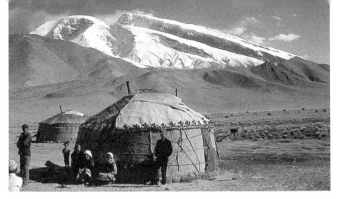

Kirghiz akoi in front of Muztagh Ata

CHAPTER 1

Adapting to High Altitude

As you gain altitude the air becomes thinner, the barometric pressure falls, and less oxygen is available. Imagine traveling in a modern pressurized airplane at 29,000 feet (8800 meters). If the cabin were to suddenly lose pressure, so that the air inside was at the same pressure as the air outside, unless you were breathing supplemental oxygen you would lose consciousness in about four minutes and die. However, Everest, at the same altitude, has been climbed many times without supplemental oxygen. What's the difference between the two scenarios? A gradual process in the body called *acclimatization*, during which the body slowly gets used to the lower levels of oxygen in the air. Individuals who have acclimatized properly are able to climb unassisted to altitudes as high as Everest and survive for short periods of time.

What happens as your body gets used to less oxygen?

The end result of acclimatization, which occurs over a period ranging from days to weeks, is that the body adapts to the increasingly rarefied air and delivers the necessary amounts of oxygen to the cells. The examples in this book describe the changes occurring in a person who is born and raised near sea level and who occasionally goes to altitude. Those who are born and raised at high altitudes, such as in the Himalaya or the Andes, may not experience these specific changes. But if you live at lower altitudes, such as at 5000 feet (1520 meters) or more, you will find it easier to tolerate higher altitude because you have already acclimatized, to some extent.

The following analogy is helpful in understanding the process of acclimatization. Imagine a freight train delivery system. Your blood vessels are the tracks. The train (your blood) is propelled by a locomotive (the heart) and has boxcars (your red blood cells) carrying a cargo (oxygen). The train's cargo is filled by a loader (your lungs) and empties its load at the factory (muscles, heart, brain, and other tissues), where the cargo is needed. Not all the cargo arriving at the loader at any one time is loaded. Much is sent back out, only to arrive again.

As an individual gains altitude, less and less cargo arrives at the loader each minute, but the demand at the factory remains constant. What does your body do? It responds by increasing the speed of the loader (makes the lungs breathe faster), increasing the speed of the train (makes the heart beat faster), and increasing the number of boxcars (makes more red blood cells). In this chapter, we will look at this process in detail.

In this book, *low altitude* is defined as 7000 feet (2130 meters) or lower; *intermediate altitude* extends to 12,000 feet (3660 meters); *extreme altitude* is above 18,000 feet (5490 meters). The term "high altitude" encompasses the ranges of intermediate and extreme altitude.

BREATHING ADAPTATION

The most important adaptation you'll notice as you ascend is the need to breathe more often. For example, when you drink from a water bottle you may need to stop in the middle to take a breath. Or you may need to stop talking to breathe. In general you'll breathe more both when active and when resting.

Each individual responds to the lowered oxygen at altitude differently. Some people breathe more often than others. Using the train analogy, if there is less oxygen in each loader (your lungs), then you will make the loader work faster in order to get the oxygen you need. Your capacity to do this can be decreased by taking sleeping pills or increased by drugs, such as acetazolamide, that signal the loader to work faster. While some people advise using different techniques to increase the rate of breathing, simply breathing more, consciously or not, is the most important factor. Generally speaking, most world-class altitude climbers increase their breathing at altitude more than superb marathon runners do, likely due to different genetic makeup. However, psychological drive can make up for differences in the capacity to breathe at altitude. An excellent example is provided by Peter Habeler and Reinhold Messner, the first two people to climb Everest without oxygen. One has a brisk rapid breathing response to altitude, while the other doesn't.

PULSE INCREASE

Just as your respiration rate increases as you climb higher, your resting pulse increases during the first few days at altitude. If there is less oxygen in each boxcar (red blood cells), then the train's locomotive (your heart) will have to go faster to unload the same amount of oxygen at the factory as before.

It's a good idea to measure your pulse rate each day when you are resting and relaxed at an altitude destination. Taking your pulse immediately after awakening in the morning is best, but you can also take it before you go to sleep.

As you become more acclimatized, you will notice that your pulse drops, and there is less pounding in your chest. This can be a sign that your body is responding well to altitude. Drugs for angina or for high blood pressure may limit this response, in which case taking your pulse won't be a useful way to judge what is happening. Such drugs include beta blockers (atenolol, metoprolol, propranolol, timolol), calcium channel blockers (verapamil, diltiazem, nifedipine), and digoxin.

URINARY RESPONSE

The body experiences *diuresis* at altitude; that is, you urinate more and lose fluids. If the freight train represents your blood, then diuresis means getting rid of non-cargo carrying cars, such as empty flatbeds. Diuresis occurs when you sleep at 10,000 feet (3050 meters) or higher and is thought to occur through stretch receptors in the heart. When diuresis takes place, you will have to get up one or two times in the middle of the night to urinate, and you can lose up to 2 percent of your body weight in water. If it doesn't happen, be more wary of altitude illness; this doesn't mean that you will get altitude illness, but you are more susceptible.

BLOOD RESPONSE

At altitude the blood thickens, a process that takes a month or more to complete. Actually, in the first few days your blood gets thicker because of the diuresis and associated fluid loss. Later it becomes thicker because the body makes more red blood cells to carry the oxygen. Using the freight train analogy again, if each train adds more boxcars (red blood cells), it can carry more cargo (oxygen). But this can be a problem if there are too many boxcars, each carrying a small payload. The train (blood) then becomes too heavy and can't travel as fast or as efficiently; that is, your blood becomes too thick.

Thick blood can clot easier, or it can sludge and cause problems in delivering oxygen where it is needed. Inactivity, such as being confined in a tent for a few days by a storm, can increase the risk of developing a clot that could migrate. For example, blood clots in the legs can migrate to the lungs and become life-threatening. Migrating clots may be a more common problem than previously thought and could explain the sudden, rapid deterioration of people high up in the mountains. If caught in such a situation, force yourself to exercise. Go outside if possible. If you can't get out, do isometrics or undertake make-work projects.

It's been suggested that blood should be thinned by removing some of the extra red blood cells, but this doesn't appear to work. Others recommend taking drugs such as aspirin, which makes the blood less sticky and less likely to clot. There are no studies of this at altitude. In some cases, thinning the blood could result in problems such as increased bleeding from an injury or a stomach ulcer. Opinions on whether people should take aspirin at altitude are divided; it may make sense for those spending relatively long periods of time at extreme altitudes (above 18,000 feet or 5490 meters), but its effectiveness is not certain (most things aside from death and taxes are uncertain). I recommend aspirin for people who will spend more than a week at altitudes above 15,000 feet (4570 meters), especially if facing periods of inactivity. If you decide to take aspirin, one 325 mg tablet (or even a baby aspirin tablet) every other day is probably adequate.

CHANGES DURING SLEEP

Most people at altitude experience some difficulty in falling asleep. Sleep may be irregular, and some individuals may wake up breathless at altitudes above 8000 feet (2440 meters). But sleep irregularities are much more common at altitudes above 15,000 feet (4570 meters). In the tent you may hear your companions' breathing increase and become loud, decrease after a minute or two and become very quiet, almost imperceptible, or even cease, and then start up again. This pattern is called *periodic breathing*. Sometimes before breathing starts up again, the sleeper may awake, startled. This occurs during the initial phase of rapid breathing when the body builds up oxygen in the brain, and the need to breathe diminishes. Just before the respiration becomes almost imperceptible, the brain, starved for oxygen, wakes up the sleeper to breathe! Periodic breathing often gives people anxiety, and some may wish to abandon their trip. It is normal, however, and diminishes with acclimatization. Sleeping pills will make you breathe less, and as a result, less oxygen is delivered to the tissues—not a desirable state of affairs. Don't take sleeping pills, sedatives, or most tranquilizers, all of which have the same effect. Better ways to improve the quality of sleep are described in chapter 4.

HIGH ALTITUDE DETERIORATION

People don't permanently live above 16,500 feet (5030 meters) or so for good reason: the body doesn't adapt well. The longer you stay at altitudes above 16,500 feet, the more you deteriorate physically, mentally, and emotionally. Some altitude researchers believe there is long-standing brain damage that occurs after staying above 16,500 feet for extended periods of time. In the 1920s plenty of climbers went on expeditions to Everest and to altitudes of 28,000 feet (8530 meters) without oxygen, stayed at extreme altitude for considerable periods of time, and then led productive intellectual lives. I wouldn't suggest you make your decision to avoid altitude activities because of the fear of brain damage.

OPTIMUM PERIOD FOR ACCLIMATIZATION

Acclimatizing to avoid altitude illness takes less time than acclimatizing to maximize performance at high altitude. There is no hard and fast formula for the best way; it varies with each person for every exposure. To avoid altitude illness one scheme would be to increase the sleeping altitude by 1000 feet (300 meters) each night above 10,000 feet (3050 meters). While ascending, take a break every two to three days by sleeping at the same altitude as the previous day. You can also average the process and ascend 750 feet (230 meters) a day. To make an alpine-style ascent of an 8000-meter (26,250-foot) mountain, three weeks spent at altitudes around 19,685 feet (6000 meters) might be enough, although for some, it might be too short a period and for others, too long. For a 6000-meter (19,685-foot) trekking peak, seven to ten days of acclimatizing seems reasonable.

For those making journeys to intermediate altitudes, plan to arrive a day or two early, and take it easy at first. If you will be sleeping at an altitude of 10,000 feet (3050 meters) or so, sleep at a lower altitude the day before instead of making an abrupt ascent from your base elevation. Those coming from sea level to ski in Colorado or Utah might consider spending the night in Denver. Follow the rule of "climb high, sleep low"—meaning climb as high as you can during the day, but descend and sleep at the same elevation or a little higher than the night before. If you are not feeling well, don't raise your sleeping altitude at all. Exertion should be done to moderation; don't overexert in the first few days.

Trial and error is the best way to discover your pace of acclimatizing. Don't rely on being able to repeat the acclimatization strategy with age. Some of those who went the highest fifty years ago are now quite limited in altitude tolerance, while others have limited exercise capacity.

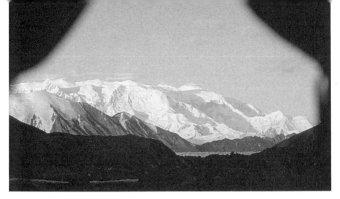

North wall, Mount Logan

CHAPTER 2

What is Altitude Illness?

It is helpful to define the terms *disease* (the opposite of ease or lack of ease), *syndrome*, and *illness* based on the biomedical model. Disease, as used here, describes entities that are disorders of physiological or psychological function. An example of a disease is the common cold, which results from an infection by one of a group of cold viruses. A cold characteristically produces a runny nose, cough, sore throat, and so forth in its victims. As of yet there are no commonly agreed upon diseases of altitude that we understand in the same detail as the common cold.

By contrast, illness can be defined as a state in which an individual feels unwell. By this definition, altitude illness comprises all the problems associated with not feeling well at altitude.

The term syndrome refers to an association of *symptoms*

(what the patient feels or complains about) and *signs* (what the health-care practitioner sees, feels, listens to, or measures) that occur together more often than would be expected by chance. AIDS (acquired immune deficiency syndrome) was originally used to describe such a group of symptoms or signs. AIDS is now recognized as an end point on a spectrum of disease caused by infection with the HIV virus. All of the illnesses of altitude—*acute mountain sickness* (AMS), *high altitude pulmonary edema* (HAPE), and *high altitude cerebral edema* (HACE), among others—are currently considered syndromes. Are all of the altitude illnesses really one disease with different manifestations, such as HIV infection, or are they different? The answer is unknown at present. Eventually, they may all represent one disease, like symptomatic HIV infection.

Sickness can be defined as a role society bestows upon an individual. This individual's behavior is characterized by some deficit in physical or mental function. Calling acute mountain sickness (AMS) a sickness means that altitude savants (the society in question) have grouped people with certain symptoms and signs together, thinking these people may exhibit facets of a single disease that is not yet well understood.

The point at which you feel the altitude (meaning that you sense a difference in functioning because of the altitude) varies with the speed of ascent and with your individual condition on a particular journey. Some people will feel the altitude at 6000 feet (1830 meters), most will feel it by 10,000 feet (3050 meters), and all will by 15,000 feet (4570 meters). Serious altitude illnesses such as HAPE or HACE can occur at altitudes around 10,000 feet (3050 meters), or even lower in some people, but are more common at higher altitudes. The likelihood of HAPE or HACE occurring will depend on how fast you ascend, your past history of adapting to altitude, and other factors that are less well understood.

It may be useful to consider altitude illness that occurs up to 18,000 feet (5490 meters) as altitude illness of acclimatization. Above this, altitude illness occurs as a part of a stay at extreme altitude where the physiology may be somewhat different than at more modest elevations. Higher, anything goes. It is much harder to study sick individuals above 18,000 feet, and our knowledge, for the most part, is based on reports rather than firsthand observation.

The syndromes of altitude illness will be described with the most common first. In the glossary, you'll find the clinical definitions agreed upon at the hypoxia meetings held at Lake Louise. A schema for diagnosis is presented in chapter 4.

ACUTE MOUNTAIN SICKNESS

AMS is the most common form of altitude illness and occurs in 20 to 70 percent of altitude sojourners. In its mild form, it feels like a hangover. AMS often occurs around 8000 feet (2440 meters) or higher but can occur at even lower altitudes. The most common *symptom* is a headache that responds to simple pain medicine, such as aspirin, acetaminophen (paracetamol), ibuprofen, or naproxen. In addition, at least one of the following symptoms is present: nausea, vomiting, lack of appetite, dizziness or lightheadedness, sleeplessness, and fatigue or weakness. AMS comes on one to three days after arrival at altitude and lasts about the same time, especially if the sleeping altitude is not raised. In a few individuals it can persist longer. Be more wary of symptoms that come on during the day while ascending, in contrast to those that manifest themselves after arrival at altitude. They may indicate more serious problems. Be wary of moderate symptoms of altitude

Table 1 Altitude Illness

Altitude Illnesses	How Common (approx. percentage)			Common Altitude of Occurrence (feet/meters)	Common Symptoms	Treatment	Other Treatment	Mortality Rate
	Trekkers to Everest Base Camp	Climbers on Mount Rainier	Climbers on Mount McKinley					
Acute Mountain Sickness (AMS) Mild	50	70	65	10,000/3050	like a hangover	don't raise sleeping altitude	simple pain medicines, acetazolamide	0
Severe	2	0	2 to 4	15,000/4575	difficulty coordinating	descend immediately	hyperbaric bag, oxygen, acetazolamide dexamethasone	low if treated quickly
High Altitude Pulmonary Edema (HAPE)	1 to 2	0	3	14,000/4270	extreme shortness of breath	descend immediately	hyperbaric bag, nifedipine oxygen	low if treated quickly
High Altitude Cerebral Edema (HACE)	0.05	0	0.5	15,000/4575	poor coordination progresses to extreme lethargy and coma	give dexamethasone, descend immediately	hyperbaric bag	higher than for HAPE

sickness, where the victim usually vomits a time or two, has a headache that cannot be relieved by the usual pain medicines, and becomes very short of breath during mild exertion.

Severe AMS can be life-threatening. It is characterized by altered balance and muscular coordination (called *ataxia* by the cognoscenti and those clinically inclined). This is the hallmark of severe AMS and may represent the earliest stage of its progression or potential progression to cerebral edema. Measure it by the *tandem walking test,* also called the drunk test or the state trooper test (see chapter 4, section III). The victim may fumble, show poor coordination, and experience an altered mental state in which he or she is not thinking clearly, be confused or disoriented, and seem unaware of surroundings and external events. Such a person may be angry, combative, lethargic or very sleepy, or incomprehensible. Some victims have been observed to be euphoric! Extreme shortness of breath with almost any activity can sometimes be observed.

It may be difficult to distinguish severe AMS from fatigue, stress, or dehydration. Also, conditions such as heat illness, exhaustion, infections such as sinusitis or malaria, and carbon monoxide poisoning from cooking inside a snow-covered tent or snow cave may also be the cause for the above-described symptoms.

Significant exercise upon arrival to altitude, by itself, predisposes people to AMS, as does younger age. Being female is not protective nor is physical fitness by itself. Individuals at greater risk of AMS include those who make a rapid ascent, especially using a vehicle for part of their journey and who thus raise their sleeping altitude abruptly; those who have had AMS before; those with a recent upper respiratory infection (cold); and those who gain weight or retain fluid at altitude or who do not urinate excessively after arrival. Others at risk include those who don't oxygenate their blood well with altitude exposure. Blood oxygenation at altitude can be measured with a *pulse oximeter* and may predict who is more likely to have AMS, although studies are inconclusive. The utility of readings may depend on the ascent profiles so no universal recommendations can be made. Those with oximetry readings that are 5 to 10 percent less than their companions may be more likely to get AMS although those with AMS have quite a range of readings. Higher differences presage HAPE, although again this has not been well studied. For a brief exposure to altitude, pulse changes may be a better indicator of AMS than pulse oximetry, although there is considerable variability with pulse rates as well. Chronic lung disease is a risk factor for AMS as is residence at sea level compared to residence at 5000 feet (1520 meters) or higher. Obese individuals and those with sleep apnea are likely at increased risk because they don't breathe as vigorously when sleeping.

There are no current tests that can be done at sea level to reliably predict susceptibility to AMS.

HIGH ALTITUDE PULMONARY EDEMA

HAPE results from an accumulation of fluid that comes from the blood and leaks into the oxygen-exchanging air sacs of the lungs. Lack of oxygen in the air coupled with high pressure in the arteries supplying the lungs promotes this condition, and it is exacerbated by cold, exercise, and dehydration. HAPE may affect 1 or 2 percent of those going up high and commonly occurs on the second night after arrival at altitude.

Early on there may be only a slight amount of extra fluid in the lungs producing only moderate symptoms that might be indistinguishable from breathing more at altitude. More commonly the HAPE victim may awaken from sleep breathing with extreme difficulty. Unlike an individual experiencing periodic breathing, a person suffering from HAPE will not be able to catch his breath and will find it very difficult to exert himself to any extent. During the day the earliest symptom experienced may be slightly decreased exercise performance, but by itself this is usually not a helpful observation. The victim's breathing will be fast (more than thirty breaths a minute in severe cases), and he will experience severe breathlessness at rest and will be unable to catch his breath or speak in full sentences. In some cases, individuals with HAPE complain only of weakness. Many people who get HAPE will already be suffering from AMS, but perhaps half or more may not. HAPE may be more common among those exercising more, such as extreme climbers, than among less active trekkers.

As the symptoms of HAPE progress, the victim becomes incapable of any significant physical exertion or activity. The pulse is rapid—and if a person has been monitoring his resting pulse at altitude, he will notice a considerable increase. In more severe cases there will be a cough, often dry, though bubbly or productive (that is, producing considerable sputum-meters). Fever is often present; for years doctors diagnosed this condition as pneumonia that failed to respond to antibiotics. As HAPE worsens the victim's color will be bluer than that of his companions (compare the color of lips or fingernail beds in daylight), reflecting his lungs' inability to transport oxygen into the blood. This is termed *cyanosis*. If you have a pulse oximeter the oxygen saturation readings in the victim will be considerably lower than in others who are not afflicted. In rare circumstances HAPE may be accompanied by HACE.

Those who are experienced in listening to the lungs may hear rales (crackles) when pressing the ear tightly against the chest wall; a stethoscope isn't necessary. They may be detected first by listening at the level of the right nipple below the armpit. Hearing these sounds in the absence of other symptoms is not helpful, as many people have crackles at altitude, but crackles are not present in the normal person after several deep breaths. Individuals affected by HAPE may also complain of chest tightness or congestion.

HAPE rarely occurs at altitudes below 8000 feet (2440 meters). So-called subclinical HAPE, a mild undetectable disease, may be more common than previously thought. Young adult males seem to be more susceptible, perhaps because they expose themselves more to the risks of the syndrome by overexerting and having a high rate of ascent. HAPE can affect residents of high altitudes when they return to high altitude after descending to an elevation below 8000 feet (2440 meters). It is more likely to affect both males and females below twenty years of age and is called reentry or resident reascent HAPE. HAPE was thought to be more common in children, although this is likely due to high altitude resident children reascending to altitude, rather than low altitude children going high.

HAPE has been thought to occur after staying at altitude for a considerable time after which acclimatization should have occurred, and many people die without the true cause of death being determined. Blood clots migrating from the legs to the lungs can be fatal. And a hole in the heart (termed a *patent foramen ovale*), normally present only during fetal growth, might open at altitude and allow clots to pass to the brain, causing a rapid demise.

The fluid in the air sacs likely results from a lung leak, rather than a lung injury. Thus if a person recovers quickly so there is no lung injury, is prudent about reascent, and takes medicine to prevent HAPE's recurrence, it may be possible to ascend again successfully.

HAPE is a serious condition, which can have a high fatality rate if untreated. Even if treated, some people will still die, especially if appropriate treatment was begun late in the illness. Once HAPE comes on, it can rapidly progress to death. Total recovery, however, is quite possible with the only consequence being a predisposition to a recurrence on revisiting high altitude destinations.

Risk factors for HAPE include prior HAPE, obesity, and the rare absence of a right pulmonary artery. Those who have a marked elevation of pressure in the arteries supplying the lungs with altitude exposure are more susceptible, but routine measurements of this are not available nor has this been done on sufficient numbers of people to establish its utility.

There seems to be a propensity for people who have previously experienced HAPE to want to taste forbidden fruit again! In the Alps, for example, there is a surfeit of subjects who have had HAPE and who are willing to go up high and test another therapy. Others just enjoy the heights. If you have had HAPE before, please follow the preventive guidelines in chapter 3.

HIGH ALTITUDE CEREBRAL EDEMA

HACE, more rare than HAPE, is related to severe AMS. HACE is believed to be caused by swelling in the brain, as the organ gets waterlogged from dilation of its oxygen-starved blood vessels. Younger people have more brain in the skull and less space to accommodate the swelling and therefore may be more susceptible. People who experience significant head injuries at altitude may also be at greater risk of HACE. The earliest sign of HACE is ataxia, or loss of balance and muscular coordination, as determined by the tandem walking test (see chapter 4, section III). They may appear mildly drunk. Ataxia or severe lassitude may remain the only sign for a period of time; coma may rapidly follow. An *altered mental status* or decreased mental functioning is usually present and will often progress, if untreated, to coma and death. Other symptoms can include hallucinations, weakness or numbness on one side of the body, blurred vision, slurred speech, inability to talk, or nonsensical talk. The course of development may range from a few hours to a day or two. A headache is almost universal; nausea and vomiting are common. In addition, symptoms of HAPE may often be present. When combined with HAPE, HACE may occur at lower altitudes. In rare cases, when victims ascend rapidly and exert significantly, HACE may develop suddenly, especially at extreme altitudes without a progression from AMS.

HACE is serious, with a high mortality rate if untreated, and has occurred at altitudes as low as 10,000 feet (3050 meters). Once a victim is unconscious, the prognosis becomes less favorable, sometimes even with appropriate treatment. Symptoms can clear quickly with descent but sometimes may persist for days, especially if the victim is in a coma. Ataxia may be the last symptom that goes away. Among those who recover, a small number can have evidence of permanent neurological injury, but some experts ascribe this damage to other conditions.

HACE may be more common among certain subgroups,

such as pilgrims ascending to high altitude for spiritual purposes.

HIGH ALTITUDE EDEMA

High altitude edema or swelling of the hands, face, and ankles is common, affecting perhaps one in five of those trekking to 14,000 feet (4270 meters). Twice as common in women as in men, it is also more frequent in those with AMS. Perhaps a third of cases occur in those without AMS. Exercise may contribute to the development of swelling. Not serious by itself, it should alert the victim and others to look at other more perilous forms of altitude illness, including severe AMS and HAPE, which are associated with fluid leaking into tissues.

HIGH ALTITUDE RETINOPATHY

High altitude retinopathy (also called high altitude retinal hemorrhage or HARH) refers to changes in the retina of the eyes, in which there is bleeding and other pathology. Usually this is not apparent to the victim or his companions. But if the changes occur in the macula, a part of the retina where the vision is most sensitive, the victim will notice a loss of sharp vision. Common in people going above 15,000 feet (4570 meters), and almost universal above 26,250 feet (8000 meters), the condition clears with descent. Slow ascent may be protective. Although considered rare at moderately low altitudes, it has been reported in combination with HAPE at ski resorts in people who briefly ascend to 11,220 feet (3420 meters). Further ascent on that trip is not advised for people who have experienced bleeding in the macula or any visual changes with HARH.

HIGH ALTITUDE SYNCOPE

Syncope, a medical term denoting a brief loss of consciousness, is called a "fainting" by laypeople. Some healthy people after arriving at altitude may stand up after eating or drinking some alcohol and faint. They normally recover quickly without further problems and do not faint again. This fainting spell may be due to blood pooling in leg veins coupled with a slow pulse that decreases blood flow to the brain. Make the victim comfortable and raise his legs above the heart.

Other conditions may cause *high altitude syncope* and require medical attention. If a person faints long after arrival at altitude, this condition warrants investigation. Making decisions for treatment in this circumstance is dependent on knowing more about the health of the individual who has fainted and requires considerable clinical judgment. The myriad causes of syncope are beyond the scope of this book.

HIGH ALTITUDE FLATUS EXPULSION

HAFE, increased intestinal gas production at altitude, remains unstudied. Most flatulent people and their companions find it annoying. Some individuals alternate burps and farts with each step up. Swallowing extra air while gasping for breath may be a factor. HAFE does not result in serious harm.

HIGH ALTITUDE COUGH

Mountaineer tales are replete with accounts of incessant coughs that keep climbers awake at night and lead to cough-related rib fractures. Coughs at altitude are common and not necessarily related to HAPE. High altitude bronchitis has been proposed as a syndrome. Activation of lung stretch receptors is implicated, but there is considerable disagreement as to how coughs are produced.

Possible causes for altitude cough include the dry air at altitude that requires plenty of energy to warm and humidify, especially given the higher breathing rates necessary for survival coupled with mouth breathing. Considerable body water is used to humidify the air you breathe in, while the heat loss in humidification can stimulate cough. Subclinical HAPE may contribute to a cough, although coughs continue to be common up high after prolonged residence and adequate acclimatization when HAPE is less likely. Upper respiratory infections (colds) are common at altitude, and coughing sensitivity is greater after such colds and may persist for long periods of time as at sea level. Finally, there may be other body chemicals released at altitude that increase the cough reflex sensitivity to cold and dry air.

OTHER SYMPTOMS AND CONDITIONS AT ALTITUDE

Since almost any condition except barotrauma and the bends from diving can occur at altitude (not to exclude that possibility when diving in high altitude lakes), this section has to be limited. Conditions that are common at sea level are likely to be common at altitude. Examples that have been reported in medical literature are mentioned here, just to underline that significant illnesses besides altitude illness occur up high. Although an illness at altitude is likely to be altitude illness, many other conditions can be present there too. Reading this may provoke fear of going to altitude, but we are probably exposed to worse risks at home.

A facial nerve or Bell's palsy might mimic HACE, but there are no mental status changes. Such people have an asymmetric smile and trouble closing an eyelid. Other localized nerve abnormalities, such as a lazy eye and double vision, can occur and can sometimes last for months. People can lose vision entirely in one eye or both or have a noticeable blind spot. A number of people have reported abrupt loss of memory—not knowing where they are, what time or day it is, or recalling other events they should know. They have no ataxia or other signs of altitude illness. Such a condition more commonly occurs at sea level, and the severe confusion can last minutes to hours and be followed gradually by complete recovery except for memory of the event. It is probably due to some temporary limitation of blood flow to the brain and is more common at sea level in older people. But the relative lack of oxygen at altitude may contribute to younger people experiencing it up high.

Individuals can similarly become delirious at altitude, perhaps brought on by the low oxygen levels. Such people are usually evacuated, because it is difficult to rule out HACE. They can experience psychiatric problems such as anxiety and panic attacks at altitude, especially since they may find themselves in insecure environments. Poor judgment or suicidal tendencies can result in overdoses from various drugs (prescription and other) they may be taking. While successfully carrying out a suicide attempt using many modern psychoactive drugs is difficult at sea level, little is known of the effects of low oxygen on drug overdose suicide attempts up high.

Brain tumors can first become symptomatic at altitude, presumably because of swelling in the brain. Similarly, people who have gone for years without a seizure may experience one at altitude. Seizures have occurred in individuals drinking too much water. There are reports of people having difficulty speaking for as long as a few hours—a transient finding called *expressive aphasia.*

Migraine headaches can occur with their sometimes-bizarre features that might lead many to suspect HACE. It would be very unusual for a migraine headache to appear for the first time in someone at altitude. The headaches of AMS may have features similar to migraines that make the diagnosis difficult. HACE can be confused with encephalitis (a brain inflammation), out-of-control diabetes, or profound electrolyte abnormalities associated with dehydration. People can faint from dehydration or other causes that are common at low altitudes.

People do have strokes and stroke-like attacks with neurological findings at altitude. One difference with such victims is that they are usually younger and without the typical cardiovascular risk factors seen near sea level. Such individuals can have one-sided weakness, numbness, or paralysis that usually resolves over the course of several hours. If coupled with a headache, the condition could be a migraine. Subsequent studies on return to sea level usually do not demonstrate any pathology. Bleeds around the brain may be more common at altitude because of increased blood flow in the brain, especially in those known to have abnormalities of cerebral vessels. Such subarachnoid bleeds may mimic HACE although the onset is usually much more abrupt.

The risk of strokes and such attacks may be increased with dehydration and the ability of the blood to clot easier. People with previously unknown clotting disorders might have such conditions strike at altitude for the first time. One climber had severe abdominal pain thought to be due to poor blood flow in an intestinal artery because of a preexisting clotting disorder.

Everest summiters and other successful high altitude climbers have experienced sudden death, presumably of cardiac causes, years later at altitude. Heart attacks have occurred at extreme altitude in young people who had never previously experienced cardiac symptoms. In one such case, strenuous exertion coupled with the altitude might have triggered a spasm in a heart artery producing the attack.

Certain constellations of symptoms are rarely attributed to altitude illness. Back and neck pain, urinary symptoms (except frequent urination from drugs that act as diuretics or from altitude exposure), and diarrhea come to mind. So while many instances of sickness at altitude represent altitude illness, you can't count on it and need to exercise good judgment.

If the above-described symptoms occur at altitude, oxygen and descent as discussed in treatment (see Chapter 5) are always recommended.

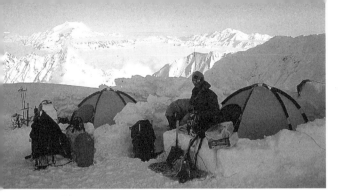

East Ridge, Mount Logan

CHAPTER 3

Preventing Altitude Illness

Altitude illness can be avoided by ascending slowly and by raising the sleeping elevation gradually. How fast is slow enough is an individual phenomenon, and the rate that worked for an individual on one trip may not work on the next. As suggested earlier, when traveling above 10,000 feet (3050 meters), try not to raise the sleeping altitude more than 1000 feet (300 meters) a night. This guideline may be too slow for some, and too fast for others. A common strategy is to climb high during the day but descend to sleep at an altitude not more than a thousand feet above where you slept the night before. Don't overexert. For every three days above 10,000 feet (3050 meters), add an extra day at the previous night's sleeping altitude to the schedule. Arrange the itinerary to acclimatize slowly. Some people, no matter how hard they try, seem to hit a brick wall at a certain elevation and cannot go higher.

When you take enough time to acclimatize, you lessen the risk of developing serious altitude illness while increasing your performance and enjoyment in high altitude activities.

In planning your trip, consider the ascent profile, that is the days and altitudes reached and sleeping altitude. Keep the rate below what would produce altitude problems in the most susceptible member of your group. The higher the final altitude and the longer the time spent at that altitude, the more cautious your ascent profile should be. Where there are large unavoidable altitude gains, plan a day or two of rest afterward. Choose a route where there is the possibility of a rapid descent (3000–6000 feet, 1000–2000 meters) should it be necessary. Sometimes mountain passes or long, level traverses can make this problematic. Consider alternative routes in such circumstances.

Mountaineers and climbers are risk takers of a different sort than the more casual skier, hiker, or trekker. The fatality rate on the highest Himalayan climbs approaches 3 percent. Nevertheless such climbing appears to be an acceptable "risk factor" to a subset of the mountaineering population. Some exhibit a "do or die" mentality and consider altitude illness an occupational hazard along with objective hazards. They may not heed the cautions about slow ascent in this book and be eager to try pharmacotherapy to help achieve summits. The great Himalayan climbers are very conscious about acclimatization and listen to an inner sense resulting from experience to determine when they are ready to go higher.

Climbers and others going to high altitudes may wish to "preacclimatize" in a hypobaric chamber, a device most often found at research military bases, but few will have access to such resources. It is preferable to use a "natural chamber"— spend time at an altitude destination nearer to home before departure for the high one. Spend as much time as you can in the natural chamber to benefit from the residual acclimatization effect that lasts from a few days up to a month or more. Obviously, the higher the natural chamber and the longer you stay, the greater the benefit. Such preacclimatization may allow a faster ascent later. I am often asked about how long the effect lasts and can only say it varies.

Those contemplating an alpine-style ascent of a major mountain usually spend considerable time acclimatizing at the base camp and make daily ascents to monitor the effectiveness of their performance at altitude. Some climbers use a tandem strategy, climbing a high peak expedition style with plenty of time for acclimatization and maximizing performance. They then do another climb, alpine style, shortly after.

Does hydration prevent altitude illness? By itself, probably not, but increasing your water intake is a vital factor in promoting well-being. The altitude environment is usually a dry one. Living and exercising there promotes increased water loss. If you take a diuretic such as acetazolamide to prevent altitude illness, you will urinate more and water loss will be increased. Therefore drinking more fluids is necessary.

Recommending that you increase your water intake to prevent altitude illness may seem paradoxical when the syndromes of altitude illness appear to result from too much water in the brain and lungs. But the fact remains that you need enough fluid in your circulatory system to keep it functioning well. One recommendation is to drink sufficient water to produce at least two bursting bladders full of urine a day. If your urine has a strong, yellow, concentrated color, you're not drinking enough. The mustard-colored snow surrounding expedition tents on high-mountain climbs attests to the difficulties of following this advice. People may not perceive their own bladder capacity accurately, so many experienced trip leaders recommend drinking at least four quarts (liters) of fluid a day. Drinking enough is easier if your water bottle is accessible and insulated if in extreme cold. A popular option today is a hydration bladder that fits into your pack and is accessed with a sipping tube. Check for adequate hydration by looking under your companion's tongue to see if saliva is pooling, or ask him to spit to see what is produced.

Too much of anything can be harmful and there are cases of over hydration with profound electrolyte abnormalities at altitude. Although very rare, constant water drinking could cause serious problems including death. Keeping warm helps lessen the rise of pulmonary artery pressures in the lungs and decreases the risk of HAPE. Temperatures fall as you gain altitude. Dehydration, cold, and the lack of oxygen at altitude are synergistic in producing HAPE. Bring clothing adequate for travel at high altitudes. Minimizing the number of times you need to stop and adjust clothing during the day will decrease fatigue. If possible, anticipate clothing changes and take off a jacket before you climb uphill, or on put insulation as soon as you stop and before you cool down. Choose clothing items that allow variable ventilation and permit adjustment and removal while moving. Garments with side and underarm zippers that allow the arms to be removed entirely from the sleeves while exercising are optimal. Being able to dress appropriately for high altitude situations comes from experience, observing others, and discussions with veterans.

Diet is important. Eat enough food, whatever is palatable, and avoid excesses of salt. Pass up alcoholic beverages at least until you are acclimatized.

Mild exercise can enhance altitude adaptation but strenuous activity could promote HAPE. Motivated athletes, who are used to exercising to exhaustion, may attempt this level of exertion up high and push beyond where normal individuals might stop. A better tactic is to increase the activity level gradually and take it easy the first few days up high. Newcomers to the heights are usually surprised at how much more slowly they function; vigorous activity before they acclimatize is usually out of the question. Fatigue will increase at altitude, so adjust the pace to ensure that you will have enough strength to finish the activity with some left for contingencies. Since a major part of adapting to altitude involves breathing more, many climbers believe that consciously doing so helps.

Out of all the drugs to be considered at altitude, acetazolamide (Diamox) is probably the best. It can be useful in preventing altitude illness, especially AMS, and is FDA approved for this purpose (although it is not approved in Europe). Taking it makes physiologic sense as it allows you to take more breaths and speeds acclimatization. It helps the body excrete carbonic acid produced from carbon dioxide, which is a by-product of your metabolism. In the freight train analogy, acetazolamide makes the loader (lungs) work faster. It is recommended for people flying or driving to altitude on tight schedules and for climbers who need to raise their sleeping altitude by 2000 feet (610 meters) or more when above 10,000 feet (3050 meters). Individuals who have had altitude illness on previous occasions may also be helped by it. There have been few reports of HACE in people who have taken acetazolamide, but this is not to suggest that it prevents it. I do not, however, recommend it for the average person traveling from near sea level to altitude in the U.S. mountain states for a brief ski vacation.

The best dose to use is controversial. If you are ascending quickly (motorized transport) from sea level, 250 mg two or three times a day is advised. If you are ascending slowly from an intermediate altitude, between 6000 feet (1830 meters) and 10,000 feet (3050 meters), 125 mg (break a 250 mg tablet in half) twice a day may be sufficient. Take the first dose before you begin ascending. A smaller dose produces less water loss through urination and causes fewer side effects. Stop taking it after one or two days at the high altitude site. Commonly reported side effects include tingling in the fingers, toes, and around the lips; frequent urination (it acts as a diuretic); and a flat taste when drinking carbonated beverages. If you're planning to use it, consider experimenting with a few test doses a couple weeks before your trip to monitor reactions and any side effects. There are no data on its use in children, but you could try a dose of 2–5 mg/kg twice a day in children. It would be best to consult a trusted doctor before the trip.

Acetazolamide is a sulfa drug and should not be taken by those who have had allergic reactions to it. Many people who think they are allergic to antimicrobial sulfa drugs have actually had an adverse reaction to them. Those experiencing adverse reactions can tolerate other sulfa drugs such as acetazolamide or the commonly prescribed diuretic furosemide. But death due to a single oral dose of acetazolamide has been reported. If you have a sulfa allergy, discuss with your doctor whether it is safe for you to take acetazolamide. Acetazolamide is also not advised for breast-feeding or pregnant women. I have included one reference (Lee et al. 2004) in the bibliography that might guide decision making regarding allergies to acetazolamide.

Dexamethasone, a potent corticosteroid, prevents altitude illness but doesn't aid acclimatization. Because of steroidal side effects, the possibility of altitude illness when use is discontinued, and the fact that it does not aid acclimatization, dexamethasone is only recommended for those who arrive at high altitude by aircraft to do rescue work. The dose is 4 mg every six hours; combine it with acetazolamide and don't take it for more than five days. Like acetazolamide, it is not advised for breast-feeding or pregnant women.

Some climbers use dexamethasone at extreme altitudes on summit day. Many people report feeling bad while taking it or after stopping it, others sense euphoria. One climber reported feeling weak, lethargic, and depressed for a month after taking dexamethasone, a marked contrast from his other altitude trips.

Studies on the herb Ginkgo biloba to prevent AMS are conflicting. The effect, if noticeable, is small from a dose of 80–120 mg twice a day, beginning five days before ascent and on the summit day. If it works, it may be most effective with moderate rates of ascent. Ginkgo biloba interferes with platelet activity in the blood, so its safety for those taking other drugs that have such effects is unknown. Some find that it also improves blood circulation to the hands in the cold. There is no standardization of preparations, so the active agent may or may not be present in sufficient quantities to work even moderately. Aspirin may work as well, but acetazolamide is the gold standard in preventing AMS.

Travelers who have previously had HAPE and are going to altitude can take nifedipine to lessen the chances of recurrence. Nifedipine dilates the pulmonary arteries; in our metaphor, it widens the roadway of the loader. The dose is 20 mg of the slow-release preparation every six hours or 30–60 mg of the 30 mg extended tablet once a day. Since nifedipine can significantly lower blood pressure, it is best to have your doctor instruct you in how to use this potentially hazardous drug. Slow ascent (about 500 feet per day) remains the most important advice in HAPE prevention.

One recent study demonstrates that salmeterol, an inhaled agent used for asthma, seems to prevent HAPE. Taken at three times the usual dose, it may have some effect in preventing the condition in those who are HAPE-susceptible. It could be considered in such people although there is limited experience in using it for this situation. The dose is 125 micrograms (six puffs) inhaled every twelve hours beginning the morning before ascent. Salmeterol belongs to a class of drugs called beta-adrenergic agents, and whether others of this class, such as the commonly used albuterol in the United States, may also work is unknown. I would also recommend that HAPE-susceptible individuals who are ascending to altitude and taking other medicines for prophylaxis also consider taking acetazolamide, although clinical studies in humans that demonstrate efficacy have not been done. For those who have not had HAPE before, no drug is recommended for prevention.

Be aware that individuals who are susceptible to AMS and HAPE on rapid ascent, such as via telepheriques in the Alps, have been able to successfully climb the world's highest peaks when they do so slowly, following the ascent guidelines presented above and not taking drugs for prevention. In other words, although you may have a history of problems with altitude illness, it is reasonable to expect that slow ascent alone may prevent further problems.

Behavioral characteristics may be one of the most important aspects in preventing altitude illness. Goal-oriented and driven people may be more at risk, as they will push themselves to go higher and deny symptoms of altitude illness. People traveling independently tend to stop and rest for a day when they feel ill. While those on adventure travel group trips, in contrast, may be more likely to die from altitude illness; this observation is based on data from Nepal (see Shlim and Gallie 1992). Such groups, if not carefully planned and guided, tend to stick to a preestablished itinerary, which may be too fast to allow certain individuals to acclimatize, making them more vulnerable to altitude illness. Peer pressure may push someone to ascend faster than she otherwise would, and splitting a party to accommodate a slow acclimatizer might pose logistical problems. Fixed schedules make it difficult for an individual to admit having symptoms of altitude illness for fear of slowing down the group or being left behind; as a result, the leader may hesitate or delay diagnosis. Because they have spent considerable money to reach the summit, members of extreme altitude climbs are less inclined to abandon their goal because of altitude illness; they may feel it is cheaper to try again while they're on the mountain rather than turn around and face the financial situation at another time. Formerly the root of all evil, money appears to be a risk factor for altitude illness as well. See "Evaluating Modes of Travel to Altitude" in chapter 7 to learn how to evaluate a commercial operator.

MAXIMIZING YOUR ENJOYMENT AT ALTITUDE

- Spend at least one night below 10,000 feet (3050 meters) before ascending higher.
- Raise your sleeping altitude by no more that 1000 feet (300 meters) each night above 10,000 feet (3050 meters).
- Climb as high as you like each day as long as you

follow the "sleeping altitude" rule.

- Build into the schedule a sleeping-altitude halt every 3000 feet (1000 meters).
- If you don't feel good, do not raise your sleeping altitude until you feel better.
- If you don't get better by staying at your current sleeping altitude, descend to where you first felt sick.
- Don't take a headache higher to sleep under any circumstances.
- Be especially concerned and vigilant if a headache comes on during the day's ascent and gets worse.
- Don't urinate into the wind or uphill if there is any wind.

THREE RULES TO AVOID DYING OF ALTITUDE ILLNESS (FROM SHLIM AND GALLIE 1992)

1. Learn the early symptoms of altitude illness and be willing to recognize when you—and others—have them.
2. Never ascend to sleep at a higher altitude with any symptoms of altitude illness. Anyone with symptoms of altitude illness who ascends will get worse.
3. Descend if your symptoms are getting worse while resting at the same altitude.

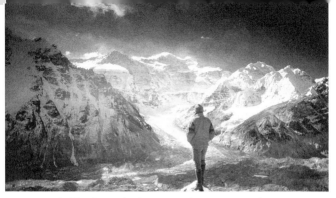

North side of Kangchenjunga, Nepal

CHAPTER 4

Diagnosing Altitude Illness

A comfortable rule used to be that if you are not feeling well at altitude, it's altitude illness until proven otherwise. Symptoms of altitude illness can be ascribed to a flu-like condition, sinusitis, dehydration, pneumonia, bronchitis, a hangover, or an ear infection, which can all present with similar symptoms. Altitude illness is the most likely cause up high, however. People commonly deny that they are suffering from altitude illness because of the effect it has on their ego, self-image, and relationship with others in the group. Such people have *attitude illness*. They need to recognize that altitude illness is not a sign of weak character or lack of conditioning.

Like almost any rule, there are exceptions. With more and more people going to great heights and some who may be beyond their prime or engaging in behaviors better avoided, various other illnesses are seen at altitude that are not altitude illness. People succumb to heart attacks, bleeds in the brain, diabetic coma, and serious infections, which makes the reasonably accurate diagnosis of altitude illness necessary. Descent, the mainstay of altitude illness treatment, is usually appropriate for them as well. But other treatment modalities may be necessary especially for life-threatening conditions such as providing sugar for a diabetic having an insulin reaction. This small book is not a treatise for every condition that may occur at altitude, just those associated with the rarified air up high; however, chapter 2 has material on other symptoms and conditions that have been reported. This chapter presents a variety of ways to diagnose altitude illness in hope that one schema will work for you.

Section I describes a systematic approach to diagnose and treat altitude illness. Like a botanical key or a decision tree, choose among pairs of statements to arrive at the appropriate presumptive diagnosis and treatment. The protocol, properly followed, should direct you to adequately treat most cases of serious altitude illness. Take notes as you go through the list.

In section II, you'll find a simpler approach to making a decision about ascending or descending. An alternative approach to these algorithms in section IV compares your functioning with that of your companions and some objective parameters. In your travel it is not slowness per se at issue. Guides report that some of their best clients are those with the wisdom to move at their own pace, which may be slow but steady. The harbinger of altitude illness is nonrecovery from tiredness or exhaustion, whatever the pace. Children are different and an approach to diagnosis for them is presented in section V.

At altitude, the lack of oxygen may affect the examiner's judgment as well. If possible, involve several people who don't

Table 2 Symptoms and Signs

Symptoms	Description	Indicator of	What to do
headache		AMS HACE	-painkillers, rest and re-evaluate in 12 hours -look for other symptoms -do not raise sleeping altitude
shortness of breath		AMS HAPE	-see if this stops with rest, if not treat for HAPE
cough		HAPE	-very common at altitude, and due to many causes besides altitude, including dry air, infections, and many other problems -needs further evaluation
extreme fatigue	having more difficulty with the activity than others	Severe AMS HAPE HACE	-check breathing and if rapid at rest, treat for HAPE -check tandem walking and if poor, treat for HACE -do not raise sleeping altitude
ataxia	lack of coordination determine by the tandem walking test	Severe AMS HACE	-descend -hyperbaric bag -oxygen -dexamethasone
altered mental status	an alternation in intellectual functioning, with emotional, attitudinal, psychologic and personality aspects	Severe AMS HACE	-descend -oxygen -hyperbaric bag -dexamethasone
diarrhea		travelers' diarrhea	-hydrate -antibiotic -consider rest day
lack of appetite		AMS HAPE HACE almost any other illness	-look for symptoms of other illnesses
feeling faint	a very difficult complaint to analyze since people can mean almost anything by it	almost any condition	-check ability to concentrate and do simple math -check tandem walking -give fluids if light-headed -consider a rest day

appear to have altitude illness in the evaluation to arrive at a better decision.

I.   A Systematic Approach to Diagnose and Treat Altitude Illness

If the suspected victim of altitude illness is not doing well or is having complaints, go through the following list sequentially from A to J. If the person is in a coma (unconscious), start with F.

A.   Are the ascent profile, signs, and symptoms compatible with altitude illness?

Talk to the suspected victim or companions about what he did on which days, how he performed those activities, at what altitude he slept, and how he felt. From his answers, you should be able to determine whether or not the problem is due to altitude, and if so, what probable altitude syndrome the victim has. If the person has been well and has descended a high pass, returned to a lower altitude, and then develops, for example, fevers, shaking, chills, and a cough, HAPE is unlikely. In a simple ski or mountain ascent, the profile is obvious, but on a Himalayan trek across several high passes or an expeditionary climb with many carries to stock high camps, there will be many variations to the altitude profile. Altitude illness rarely has a dramatic presentation, it begins insidiously and progresses. You won't see cases where an individual feels strong and energetic enough to complete a difficult ice pitch at altitude, and then suddenly collapses with serious altitude illness.

1. No. Treat the most likely cause. Descent will probably be an important part of that treatment if the condition is serious.

2. Yes. Evaluate the following:

B. Is there a headache?

1. Yes. Follow Dr. Peter Hackett's headache rule: Rest, do not ascend further, have a snack, drink fluids, and take mild pain medicine.

   a) If better and there are no other symptoms, continue with the activity.

   b) If better and there are other symptoms, continue with C. Test for ataxia (see section III, "Tests to Demonstrate Ataxia").

   c) If not better,

   (1) Test for ataxia using the tandem walking test (see section III, "Tests to Demonstrate Ataxia").

   (a) If ataxia is present, take the person down immediately (see "Descent" in chapter 5) and give dexamethasone and oxygen. The hyperbaric bag can be a temporizing step if available.

   (b) If ataxia is not present, rest at the current altitude and test again for ataxia in 6 to 12 hours.

(2) Test for altered mental status by asking the person to do simple arithmetic, such as subtracting 7 sequentially from 99 (answer is 92, 85, 78, 71, 64, etc.), or ask if he is aware of current events, specific dates, and so forth.

   (a) If there is altered mental status, check the state of hydration. If in doubt as to whether severe dehydration is the cause, rehydrate, descend, and reevaluate. Be certain the individual is not hypothermic (cold) and suffering from exposure, in which case rewarming is necessary.

   One way to check the state of hydration is to measure the pulse with the person lying down, and then have him stand up and note the rise. If it goes up twenty-five beats per minute, significant dehydration is present. Other methods include looking at the urine color (strong yellow implies dehydration), examining the lips and mouth to see how dry they appear, looking under the tongue to see if saliva is pooling, or asking the person to spit (in significant dehydration the spit is very thick if present at all).

         (*b*) If altered mental status is not present, retest for ataxia and mental status changes in 12 hours.

2.   No. If no headache, go to B.1.c. and the following:

C. Is the person short of breath?

1.   Yes. Let him rest for fifteen minutes to see if he recovers. Measure oxygen saturation if you have a pulse oximeter.

   a)   If the victim does not recover, limit further exertion and treat for HAPE by descent with limited exertion. Give oxygen if available.

     (1) If descent is not possible, have the victim rest.

        (*a*) Give a trial of the hyperbaric bag or oxygen, if available.

        (*b*) If oxygen or a hyperbaric bag is not available, give nifedipine. (See "Drugs" in chapter 5 for the protocol to use with this drug.)

   b)   If the victim recovers from his shortness of breath in fifteen minutes and there are no other symptoms, continue with the activity and recheck in a few hours.

2.   No. Check the following:

D. Does the person have a good appetite?

1.   Yes. Significant altitude illness is probably less likely but continue evaluation with E through J.

2.   No, and the person has not been urinating

copiously. Hydrate. In the absence of other symptoms or signs above, besides a mild headache, return to the previous night's sleeping altitude to sleep and rest for a day. Reevaluate in 12 hours.

3. No, and the person has been urinating copiously. Continue with the activity and reevaluate in 12 hours.

E.   Is there severely blurred or decreased vision?

1. Yes. Give the victim oxygen and/or hyperbaric therapy, if available, and descend.

2. No. Check the following:

F.   Did the person faint?

1. If the person is in a coma, treat for HACE and give dexamethasone by injection as well as the usual first-aid measures for a comatose victim. Descend as soon as possible and evacuate.

2. Yes. Ask about other health problems the person has had.

   a) If there are other causes, treat the likely ones appropriately.

   b) If there are no other causes and this happened within the first 24 hours of arrival at altitude—usually after eating, drinking, and standing—did he recover quickly (in a matter of minutes with the only treatment being leg elevation)?

      (1) No. Give oxygen, hyperbaric therapy, and descend.

(2) Yes. Check for other symptoms of altitude illness and treat accordingly. Do not sleep any higher than the night before.

3. No. Check the following:

G. Does the person have swelling of the face, hands, or feet?

1. Yes. Check for the other symptoms in this list (H to J).

   a) If other symptoms are present, treat those and reevaluate in 12 hours.

   b) If no other symptoms are present, recheck in 12 to 24 hours.

   c) If the swelling is extremely uncomfortable and a diuretic such as furosemide is available, administer as described below (see "Drugs" in chapter 5). Monitor for hydration (see B.1.c.2.*a*.).

2. No. Serious altitude illness is probably not present, given that no other symptoms in the above list exist.

H. Is the person experiencing difficulty sleeping?

1. Yes. Ask companions if periodic breathing is present.

   a) If yes or unsure, give the person 125 or 250 mg of acetazolamide at bedtime for three to four days. Do not give sleeping pills.

   b) If no, treat the companions for difficulty sleeping.

    2.   No. Reassure the person, advise against taking sleeping pills, and check the following:

I.   Is the person anxious, disoriented, irritable, or more emotional than functional?

    1.   Yes. Retest for ataxia and altered mental status and follow that protocol.

    2.   No. Continue.

J.   Get answers to the following questions:

    1.   Has the person had altitude problems before?

        a)   At what altitude, which symptoms, and what was done about it? Use this information to guide further treatment (a favorite method used by astute clinicians to treat difficult cases).

    2.   Does the person have other health problems? Oftentimes the person will have preexisting health problems that may be the cause of his discomfort. If doubtful, descent is the best recourse.

    3.   What does the victim think is going on? (Ask companions this too, it will make you a wise clinician.) Consider the answers you get in making decisions.

    4.   Is the person consuming mood-altering drugs, including alcohol? If yes, stop them from consuming those, and be prepared to deal with withdrawal symptoms. Descent may be in order.

MONITORING ALTITUDE ILLNESS

To gauge the response to your treatment, measure and record the heart and respiratory rates, list them together with the symptoms and signs, and note observation times. Include oxygen saturation if you have a pulse oximeter. Repeat the assessment frequently, for example, at intervals of 4 to 24 hours depending on the severity of the illness.

II. Simplified Decision Tree

Begin with section I, "A Systematic Approach to Diagnose and Treat Altitude Illness," to determine if the ascent profile, signs, and symptoms are compatible with altitude illness.

A. **If altitude illness is suspected, don't ascend.**

B. **Descend if you don't get better, or immediately if:**
   1. There is severe shortness of breath at rest; that is, the victim doesn't catch her breath after resting fifteen minutes.
   2. Ataxia is present (see section III).
   3. There is no improvement in the symptoms and signs while resting at the same altitude.
   4. The person is getting worse.
   5. Confusion or hallucinations are present.

C. **If you ascend with altitude illness, you will get worse.**

III. Tests to Demonstrate Ataxia

Let the subject who is having difficulty at altitude rest. Once rested, administer the tandem walking test. Draw a straight line at least 6 feet (2 meters) long on the ground or in the snow with the heel of a boot or a stick. Choose a safe level place with no rocks or debris. Demonstrate how to walk along the line, putting the heel of the foot ahead and touching the toe of the foot behind. Have the subject attempt this. Slight difficulty, using the arms for balance, is tolerable if 12 feet (4 meters) can be walked in a straight line. If the person steps off the line or falls to the ground, the test is abnormal. Assuming you do not have severe AMS yourself, your competence in doing this serves as a control to assess the potential victim. Rugged terrain may make it more difficult for both of you to accomplish the maneuver. With exhaustion, hypothermia, or mild intoxication, some loss of coordination (ataxia) can be seen, but there should be no staggering or falling.

Another test to try is the Romberg. Have the person stand, feet together, arms at the side (or held out in front), and eyes closed. If the person sways considerably, significant loss of coordination (ataxia) is present. Again, use an unaffected member of the party as a comparison.

IV. Altitude Illness in Yourself and Your Companions

A. **Symptoms or signs to look for in yourself that would lead you to suspect significant altitude illness:**
   1. Resting pulse above 110 beats per minute.
      a) Be especially wary if your pulse at

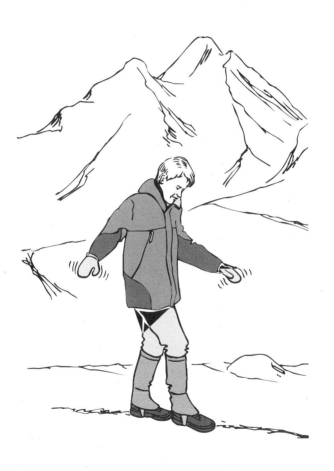

Tandem walking test

altitude goes up after having been at altitude for a while.

b) Measure your pulse in the same circumstance each time; for example, lying in a tent in the morning.

c) Your pulse may go up from caffeine or anxiety, but should not remain high after resting.

2. If you are on medicines to control the heart-beat or blood pressure, treat angina, or prevent migraine headaches (see "Pulse Increase" in chapter 1), you may not have a high resting pulse yet could still have altitude illness.

3. Marked shortness of breath at rest (after you have recovered from the activity and are breathing more than twenty times a minute).

4. Loss of appetite.

5. Great fatigue while undertaking an activity, especially if it is increasing in comparison to your companions' level of fatigue.

B. Signs to look for in your companions suggesting significant altitude illness:

1. Someone skipping meals and wanting to spend more time in the tent.

2. Change in behavior. For example, someone who:

a) Becomes quiet and retiring when he had been gregarious before.

b) Is a quiet person who becomes quieter.

c) Becomes obnoxious. You notice new difficulties in getting along with this person.

           d)   Persistently very somnolent.

3.   An individual having more trouble with an activity than his companions, especially if this is not usually the case. For example,

    a)   If trekking, this person is the most tired on arrival at the destination.

    b)   If skiing, this person is constantly falling and is the slowest.

    c)   If climbing, this person is getting much slower and is less competent when doing technical climbing.

    d)   If during a group meeting, this person becomes forgetful and loses the theme of the discussion.

C. The following methods are the best ways to confirm the suspicion of altitude illness if the signs and symptoms described above are present:

1.   Increase the victim's oxygen intake, either by having the victim descend, giving oxygen by mask, or placing the victim in a hyperbaric bag and observing the response. Descent is the preferred option.

2.   Wait at a specific altitude that is no higher than the previous night's sleeping altitude to see if the victim gets better. This is recommended only for those who have mild to moderate AMS or high altitude edema. It is not recommended for High Altitude Pulmonary Edema (HAPE) or High Altitude Cerebral Edema (HACE) when immediate descent is necessary.

V.   Diagnosing Altitude Illness in Children

Taking your children to altitude is discussed in chapter 6. If you are not doing well at altitude, this compounds the difficulty of determining if an infant or child is having altitude illness. Here are suggestions based on research.

Verbal children, three to eight years old, may not be reliable reporters of symptoms of altitude; assessing behavioral changes or irritability in children younger than three is more reliable than asking about symptoms. New environments can also produce similar changes, making a "diagnosis" more difficult. Have a high index of suspicion for altitude illness if traveling with children.

If you take children younger than three years old to altitude, the following schema may be helpful in considering whether altitude is the cause of how the child is behaving. Fussiness, an irritable state without an identifiable cause (hunger, wet diaper, injury), should be evaluated in terms of how much is present and for how long in comparison to the usual situation for that child. How well is the child eating? Is he vomiting? How active and playful is the child? Finally, does the child sleep as he would normally? Gauging color helps as well; the skin tone of a sick child may be blue or dusky or just not look right. If the child is extremely fussy and inconsolable, not eating, and not playing or sleeping, immediately descend with the child. If the child exhibits no fussiness, eats and plays normally, and sleeps well, there is less likelihood of significant altitude illness.

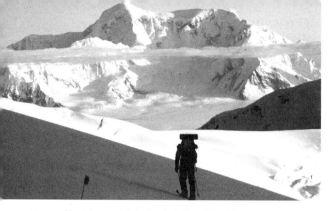

Descending King Trench in front of Mount St. Elias

CHAPTER 5

Treatment of Altitude Illness

Various methods for treating altitude illness for the nonmedical practitioner are described. Treatment for severe AMS and for presumed HAPE and HACE are given together. Treatment protocols for health-care providers in a clinical facility at intermediate altitude are outlined separately.

REST

Rest for mild to moderate symptoms of AMS may be the only treatment necessary and one that is commonly overlooked. For the more serious conditions, exerting as little as possible is vital treatment. In high Andean clinical facilities where oxygen was not available, rest has been a successful treatment under medical supervision. If physical activity is required, it should be in the direction outlined next.

DESCENT

There used to be just three rules for treating altitude illness: descend, descend, descend! This remains the gold standard of care. It is almost never a bad decision. But these days, with other treatment modalities available, it is sometimes easy to forget the gold standard, and the consequences can be fatal! Descent is usually the most appropriate treatment. The amount of descent necessary to see an improvement is generally 1000 to 3000 feet (300 to 910 meters). Make note of the altitude at which even mild symptoms first occurred, the victim's threshold of altitude illness on this occasion. Descend below this altitude after serious symptoms develop.

Altitude illness may become apparent in the afternoon when the terrain is difficult. In groups there may be confusion over who is in charge to make decisions about evacuation, especially in a trip organized from one country to another where a local agent provides the ground-based services. Make every effort to get the victim down early, relying on his own ability to walk. Don't wait for the person to stagger or become unconscious and require evacuation. If you take this advice to heart, you may need to insist on going down against the pro-testations of the sick person, who is determined to be "tough" or sometimes even the leader. Take charge, don't be polite.

When HAPE is suspected, minimize the victim's exertion. When there are no other vehicles, have the victim transported by a pack animal (horse, donkey, yak) or on someone's back. Self-descent in very early stages of HAPE is acceptable. Bad weather and hazardous terrain can stall the decision to evacuate to a lower altitude. Skilled mountaineering judgment regarding the safety of a descent must be weighed against the severity of the illness.

Increasing availability of helicopter transport, at one time common only in the Alps, is now changing the rescue capabilities for many. Satellite phones and other communication facilities in high tourist traffic areas can facilitate this. Bad weather, the desire of people to not disappoint and say "yes, the aircraft is coming," as well as equipment difficulty can make waiting at a high altitude site and not descending catastrophic. Waiting for an air rescue can take several days in many situations, while altitude illness can progress to death in hours! Faced with this situation, describe the descent route and signaling materials to those organizing the air evacuation, and then proceed with the descent and signal to make contact. If you know the frequencies used in the area to which you are traveling, carrying two-way radios can be very helpful. In some areas such as the Tibetan Plateau, aircraft may be unavailable.

Use judgment in planning a helicopter rescue. Pilots may fly in extreme conditions, and crashes are common. Don't expose others to danger for minor problems. And if you are not awaiting an air rescue, please do not signal an aircraft that may be trying to evacuate a seriously afflicted person.

The first symptom to improve with descent in HACE is usually the confusion and other alterations in mental status. The last to improve may be the loss of coordination, or ataxia.

If the sick person is not improving at least a little with descent or is getting worse, then serious altitude illness (HAPE or HACE) is probably not the only major problem. Although the coma of HACE may take some time to improve, other signs and symptoms usually demonstrate some beneficial progress. Reassess. If another condition besides altitude illness is causing the symptoms, treat that. Descent will not make the person worse.

OXYGEN

Oxygen, if available, should be given in all cases except mild or moderate AMS. There is no harm in giving oxygen at altitude. Use a mask or nasal prongs for delivery at flows of 2 to 4 liters a minute in mild HAPE or early HACE. In more severe cases, a face mask and flows of 8 to 10 liters a minute are necessary. When there is some response, decrease the dose to a level that is high enough to maintain the improvement. A pulse oximeter's readings will increase with improvement in oxygenation. If there is no response, increase the dose to 12 liters per minute. Some noticeable clinical response should occur in an hour, but sometimes it doesn't. Short-term oxygen for those with AMS and ataxia may not work quickly enough to ameliorate the loss of coordination, although other symptoms may improve. Continue the oxygen and then consider other modes of treatment. In seriously ill individuals do not delay descent in order to give oxygen. Get the person down while giving oxygen if possible.

Some altitude destinations have oxygen available for emergency use. Portable oxygen concentrators, which require a power supply, are available, and more and more facilities are powering them with solar and wind generators. At the Himalayan Rescue Association's aid posts in Phierche and Manang the use of portable oxygen concentrators has all but replaced the hyperbaric bag. Carrying bottled oxygen is possible, although weight usually limits carrying large amounts. But the advantage is that descent can be undertaken with it.

HYPERBARIC BAG

Igor Gamow, working with others, developed a portable, fabric cylinder to accommodate a victim of altitude illness. Inflated by a foot pump to produce a pressure of 2 psi (103 mm Hg) over existing air pressure, it simulates a descent of several thousand feet (thousand meters). Pump strokes about every five seconds maintain the pressure. The higher the bag is used, the greater the relative descent. Groups going to altitudes above 15,000 feet (4570 meters) to trek or climb should consider purchasing or renting one. There are currently three versions available: a U.S. model, Gamow Bag; a European, Certec Caisson; and an Australian model, PAC (Portable Altitude Chamber), which is also the most affordable. Though expensive, a bag is cheaper than a coffin!

Advantages of the hyperbaric bag over oxygen stem from its portability and sustainability. You cannot run out of air to pressurize it, so it can be used over and over to re-treat the victim or to treat others. Oxygen is bulkier and heavier, and cylinders run out. But nonvehicular methods of descent are not possible with the bag. Be sure to test the bag first as it can leak, the zipper can wear out, and the pump can malfunction. A patch, applied to the inside, can salvage a leaky bag. Compared to descent as treatment, once you use the bag and come out of it, you are still at the high altitude, which can prove fatal.

For a trekking group, carrying the bag and oxygen makes sense. For a mountaineering expedition, deciding where to store the bag can be problematic. Leaving it at higher camps may make the bag inaccessible, while keeping it lower down may make it unavailable when needed.

Someone with mild to moderate AMS might benefit from an hour or two in the bag, though this may not represent a significant improvement over just resting and using mild analgesics for 24 hours. Even if he gets better, he should be watched carefully to see if symptoms return. If symptoms are only mild, the person can stay at that altitude, but if more severe symptoms come on, descent is appropriate.

If descent is not possible, those with severe symptoms of AMS or symptoms of HAPE or HACE should be treated in the bag for four to six hours. When anything other than mild HAPE is suspected, and if the person improves, he should subsequently descend and take medicines as outlined below. A victim treated with the bag should not be removed from access to the bag until he is clearly better or has descended to below where the first symptoms of altitude illness occurred. In one documented case, an individual with severe altitude illness used the bag, improved, did not descend, and subsequently died when the bag was taken elsewhere. Use the bag for serious conditions when descent is impossible or too risky because of terrain, time, or weather.

The bag may not work as well for HAPE as it does for HACE. Patients with severe HAPE can find it very uncomfortable to lie flat in the small models, while someone with HACE may struggle. Prop up the head end of the bag on an inclined plane until the patient has experienced enough improvement to tolerate lying flat. For seriously ill patients, if you have an oxygen cylinder and delivery system, connect it to the person and place it in the bag with him. Combine drug treatment with use of the bag. If the victim is not breathing, the bag will not help. If the victim is in a coma with minimal or no gag reflex and if you have the equipment and skill to perform endotracheal intubation, the procedure may be advisable in order to protect the airway before putting the victim in the bag.

If you haven't done so already, read the instructions before putting the victim into the bag. The patient should attend to urination and defecation beforehand. Put a pee bottle, a towel, and a sleeping bag in the bag with the victim, and put the victim in the sleeping bag if conditions warrant. An oxygen delivery system can be put inside in extreme cases. If you have a pulse oximeter, connect it and attach the meter to the person so you can see it through the window. Similarly, an altimeter can help you gauge virtual descent. Explain to the victim the need to breathe normally and recommend that he pop his ears by swallowing or blowing gently against the pinched nose as the bag is inflated. Tell the victim that if the bag should suddenly deflate, he should exhale. Before closing the zipper, ask the victim to extend his arms and legs to increase the air space inside the bag to save time and effort during inflation. Once the bag is inflated, ten to twenty pumps a minute are usually necessary to maintain it and excess pressure as well as carbon dioxide buildup is relieved through a pop-off valve. Condensation around the window may make it difficult to monitor the patient. Try covering the bag (except for the window) with a sleeping bag and have the patient use the towel to wipe condensation off the window.

When the bag is used, an observer should be with the victim at all times and talk reassuringly to him. If it is cold, put the patient in a sleeping bag; if out in the hot sun, be sure to shade the bag to avoid overheating. Considerable physical effort is needed to maintain the pressure in the bag. While it may be lifesaving in buying time, it usually only postpones the need to descend. After someone with serious altitude illness improves in the bag, avoid exertion after he emerges. Some may be able to tolerate exercise, while others may quickly relapse.

For the victim, problems associated with using a hyperbaric bag include feeling claustrophobic as well as difficulty clearing his ears and sinuses with the increasing pressure. People can vomit inside and possibly aspirate especially if drowsy with decreased mental functioning. If a person vomits, get them out of the bag immediately and clear the airway.

The current models use a dry suit zipper as a seal. The European version has an outer and inner bag. The Australian features a radial zipper opening at the head making access easier together with an ability to decrease the pressure pop-off point for those experiencing difficulty clearing their ears. This relatively inexpensive model has a larger window that makes it more comfortable for those outside and inside. This unit also comes with an instruction book in Nepali. Obese individuals find it difficult to get in and out of this model because they have to slide in from the top, while it is a challenge to get tall unconscious victims into the U.S. and European models. Bag durability may limit the number of seasons they can remain functional. Valves are prone to get dirty and not seal well but can easily be blown clean. A larger version, the Gamow Tent, with an internal frame and space for two has been produced. This tent would be good for placing a healthy parent and sick child together or a critically ill patient with an attendant, but it is not widely used.

When oxygen is available, it is always preferable to a bag. However, given problems with powering oxygen concentrators and bottled oxygen supply, having a bag for backup is wise.

Gamow Bag is produced by Hyperbaric Technologies, Inc., One Sam Stratton Road, P.O. Box 69, Amsterdam, NY 12010; 518-842-3030, Fax 518-842-1031; *plewis@bretonindustries.com* and is distributed by Chinook Medical Gear, 120 Rock

Point Drive, Unit C, Durango, CO 81301; 800-766-1365, 970-375-1241, Fax 970-375-6343; *www.chinookmed.com; admin@chinookmed.com.* This company also rents bags and is a source for pulse oximeters.

Certec Caisson from Certec, Le Bourge, 69210 Sourcieux Le Mines, France, 33-74-70-3982, Fax 33-74-70-3766; *www.certec.fr/homeN.html; info@certec.fr.*

PAC manufactured by C. E. Bartlett Pty, Ltd., Ring Road, Ballarat, P.O. Box 49, Wendouree, Victoria 3355, Australia; 61 3 5339 3103, Fax 61 3 5338 1241; *www.bartlett.net.au/pac/pac.html; info@bartlett.net.au;* with distribution by Treksafe, P.O. Box 53, Repton NSW 2454, Australia; 61 66 534 241, Fax 61 2 6653 4130; *www.treksafe.com. au; pac@treksafe.com.au.* Bags can be also rented in Kathmandu (*www.bartlett.net.au/pac/pac.html*).

DRUGS

ACETAZOLAMIDE

Acetazolamide (Diamox) is recommended for treating symptoms of AMS of any degree in adults. Although unlikely to make a great difference in severe AMS, it should be taken nevertheless. The dose for mild AMS can be as low as 125 mg at bedtime to improve sleep but increase it to 250 mg, two to three times a day for moderate to severe AMS. Continue until the victim feels much better. Common side effects include numbness or tingling of the hands, feet, and area around the mouth; increased urination; nausea; and a flat taste when drinking carbonated beverages. Some individuals find the side effects unacceptable and cannot tolerate this drug. While it is safe to give to children, there is no experience in using it at altitude with this population.

For mild to moderate AMS, acetazolamide coupled with not raising the sleeping altitude may be sufficient treatment. There is no evidence that it masks altitude illness. If you take it and improve, then you are improving! In more severe situations, it is an adjunct, requiring other treatments. There is some controversy over the appropriate dose to use. I advise lower doses for mild symptoms and higher doses for more severe illness, but do not exceed 750 to 1000 mg per day.

Acetazolamide is a sulfa drug and should not be taken by those truly allergic to sulfas (see chapter 3 for allergy details). For individuals with frostbite the diuretic effect of this drug could affect circulation by producing dehydration and causing further injury especially when used in higher doses.

NIFEDIPINE

For a victim suffering from mild HAPE (capable of some physical activity) and no other altitude illness other than mild AMS, nifedipine may effectively treat the condition. He should descend until improved and then continue descent or possibly consider ascent (see below). In more severe cases, urgent descent and treatment in addition to nifedipine will be necessary. Monitor the dose and response and use judgment to adjust the dose where necessary.

Treatment with nifedipine can lower blood pressure enough to cause someone to fall or faint, so use it with caution. In one documented case, it prevented a climber from standing up in a precarious position. Even more disastrous situations can be imagined. When using this drug, avoid being in a potentially hazardous situation and have a responsible individual monitor the response.

Performing a nifedipine treatment trial for HAPE can help determine if HAPE is actually the problem. Have the victim rest quietly in a safe place and give him a 10 mg capsule of nifedipine after puncturing it several times with a pin. Instruct the victim to chew and swallow the drug; do not leave it under the tongue. If the person subsequently feels faint, have him lie down. The victim may note easier breathing in ten minutes. If the person has not become profoundly faint and is breathing better, repeat the dose in fifteen minutes. After thirty minutes and two doses, if the person's symptoms are noticeably better and he has not fainted, give 20 mg of the slow-release preparation (Adalat) every six hours. If you have the 30 mg long-acting preparation (Procardia XL) give one or two tablets a day. Maintain hydration. You can stop the drug after a few days or when symptoms have been absent for twenty-four hours.

If the person becomes severely light-headed or faints while taking nifedipine, have him lie on his back, elevate his legs to promote the return of blood to the heart, and stop giving nifedipine. When the individual is wide awake and can drink, give fluids. Don't allow him to stand unattended until he can do so without feeling light-headed and can walk unassisted. Do not give fluids by mouth to someone who is unconscious! Rely on other treatments for HAPE, especially descent, oxygen, or the hyperbaric bag.

Those with experience using a blood-pressure cuff to monitor postural changes may reduce the likelihood of overdosing someone with large amounts of nifedipine and causing adverse effects.

Another monitoring method compares pulse readings while the person is standing with pulse readings while he is lying down before and after the first dose of nifedipine. If the standing pulse is twenty points per minute more than the lying pulse and the person feels light-headed, there is a significant postural drop in blood pressure. This means the standing blood pressure is lower compared with the lying blood pressure, and the brain is being deprived of blood. Rehydrate the person and check the difference in pulse again. If the drop is less than twenty, give the first dose of nifedipine, and recheck the pulse changes lying and standing in fifteen minutes. Use pulse changes to guide further doses of nifedipine as if monitoring blood pressure.

If you have a pulse oximeter you should notice some improvement in the oxygenation readings. If not, question the diagnosis or add other treatment.

The highly motivated climber or skier vacationing at a resort might contemplate further ascent if the treatment for HAPE was successful and certain conditions can be met. People have successfully reascended after recovery from HAPE in circumstances where there was medical supervision in case problems recurred. If the illness was mild and the recovery swift and if the victim was able to rest for a time at a lower altitude, you can consider slowly reascending with responsible companions; in this situation, nifedipine is also recommended. Read the protocols for health-care providers (below) for guidelines.

The best experience with nifedipine at present is in the European Alps. There, climbers have ascended rapidly, succumbed to HAPE, and recovered quickly when they have been speedily treated with nifedipine. Reports to date in Alaska and the Himalaya, where ascent rates are usually slower, suggest

Table 3 High Altitude Drugs

Name	Use	Form	Dose	How Often	Common Side Effects	Notes
oxygen	treatment of all forms of altitude illness	cylinders by mask, or nasal prongs	1 to 12 liters a minute; begin with 6 liters for serious problems	continuously	none in the mountain setting except possibly dry mucous membranes	delivery units with tight-fitting masks and a reservoir bag
acetazolamide	prevention of AMS	250 mg tablet	1/2 to 1 tablet	twice a day or at bedtime	increased urine output; tingling of lips and extremities	do not give if allergic to sulfa drugs
	treatment of AMS		1 tablet	twice at day for treatment		
nifedipine	treatment of HAPE	10 mg capsule (pricked many times with a pin)	1 capsule chewed and then swallowed	repeat in 15 minutes	lowering of blood pressure	see text for protocol details; follow with prevention dose
	prevention and treatment of HAPE	20 mg slow-release capsule (Adalat) 30 mg extended release tablet (Procardia XL)	1 capsule swallowed / 1 or 2 tablets	every 6 hours / daily	lowering of blood pressure details / ankle swelling is commonly seen in lowlanders	see text for protocol
dexamethasone	treatment of severe AMS and HACE	4 mg tablets	1 tablet	every 6 hours	emotional problems especially after stopping the drug; depression and euphoria reported while taking it	first dose 2 tablets, stop after problem has resolved, or taper (see text)
furosemide (frusemide)	treatment of peripheral edema	40 mg tablets	1/2 to 1 tablet	once a day	can cause fainting if taken while dehydrated	stop after edema has resolved; eat potassium (bananas, pigmented fruits); drink plenty of liquids

that the response is protracted and not as dramatic. There is no central reporting scheme, so good experiences with it cannot be correlated with reports of it not working or causing serious side effects. Acetazolamide, in contrast, has been in use for more than twenty-five years and has been evaluated by several controlled double-blind trials, the gold standard of assessment. We have a better understanding of what it can and probably cannot do.

For children, there is no experience with nifedipine, but a dose of 0.25 mg/kg could be tried. And then follow with the long-acting preparation at similar doses twice a day. Consider the drug in extenuating circumstances where you can monitor the blood pressure.

DEXAMETHASONE

Dexamethasone, a corticosteroid, is recommended for treating anyone with severe symptoms of AMS and as an adjunct to the other therapies in treating HACE. Give 8–10 mg initially followed by 4 mg every six hours by mouth. There is no need to place a tablet under the tongue. If the victim is in a coma, the drug should be injected. If taken early enough in the course of the illness, it might prevent progression to more serious symptoms. In situations where it is given for days on end, consider tapering the dose (giving less each day) as improvement occurs. If someone takes this drug for what turns out not to be altitude illness and later wants to continue activity at altitude, he should only do so after stopping dexamethasone. For children, if unable to descend, try a dose of 0.5 mg/kg every six hours.

PAIN MEDICINES

The most common analgesics and NSAIDs (nonsteroidal

anti-inflammatory drugs) include aspirin (acetylsalicylic acid), acetaminophen (paracetamol), ibuprofen, and naproxen. There are myriad more available by prescription in most Western countries, but avoid Cox-2 inhibitors. They can be used for headaches and the hangover-like symptoms in usual doses.

NARCOTICS

Narcotics, including oxycodone, hydrocodone, hydro-morphone, meperidine, pethidine, morphine, and various others, should not be used at altitude as they can depress respiration. Codeine in low doses (30–60 mg) may be safer to use.

DIURETICS

When swelling of high altitude edema is severe enough to cause discomfort and limit activity, a potent diuretic such as furosemide in small doses (20 or 40 mg orally) can be taken daily. The response is usually rapid. Give plenty of fluids. If there are other symptoms beyond those of mild AMS, do not use this potentially hazardous therapy.

In cases of HACE, where rapid descent is delayed, use of diuretics such as furosemide should be considered.

ANTI-VOMITING MEDICINE

Although prochlorperazine (Compazine and other brands) would be the preferred drug because it stimulates respiration, it also can cause bizarre muscular side effects, so I would not recommend it. Promethazine is safer, though it doesn't stimulate respiration. The rectal route is the preferred way to administer any anti-vomiting medicine. Consider injecting dexamethasone and descending if vomiting is severe.

OTHER DRUGS THAT MIGHT BE EFFECTIVE
Sildenafil

Sildenafil (Viagra) belongs to a class of drugs that have gained attention for treating erectile dysfunction. The drug also reduces pulmonary artery pressure (increased pressures are the hallmark of HAPE) just as nifedipine does. There are no published studies to date of its use for this condition, nor is there FDA approval, of course. Sildenafil has been proposed to enhance exercise performance at altitude, but there are no clinical studies of its use other than by experimental subjects. I expect that more altitude-related studies may appear in the future for this class of drugs, but for the present, other therapies for which we have considerable evidence suggesting efficacy should be used. These include oxygen, rest, hyperbaric chamber, descent, and nifedipine. If you have no other drug treatment modalities available and have access to sildenafil, a person with severe HAPE could be given a dose of 50 mg every 4 hours.

Sleeping pills

Difficulty sleeping is reported by many at altitude. Reasons can be many, including periodic breathing mentioned as present at altitude. Acetazolamide is the best drug for that purpose, taken in small doses before bed. Classically, sleeping pills were advised for use at altitude, but the ones usually taken caused respiratory depression and poor performance upon awakening. There are milder, shorter-acting agents now available, such as zolpidem and zaleplon. While none have been clinically tested at altitude, some experts suggest small doses may be taken without much compromise. Temazepam (10 mg) has been studied in small numbers without apparent ill effect, but I don't advise this agent.

ADJUNCTIVE TREATMENT

Those with serious altitude illness should never be left alone. The buddy system used for underwater diving makes sense at altitude. Be sure the buddy speaks the victim's language and understands altitude illness.

Keep a written record of the victim's symptoms associated with an altitude profile, what others observed, and what was done. Send this with him when transported.

Exhibiting compassion, establishing rapport with the victim, giving reassurance, listening actively, providing non-verbal support through touching, and showing concern are as important as other therapies. Reassure the victim no matter how bleak the situation appears.

Some advocate grunt breathing or pursed lip breathing with cheeks puffed out for mild HAPE. Complications of a collapsed lung, or the induction of HACE are theoretically possible.

Some climbing doctors carry a CPAP (continuous positive airway pressure) mask, with a deflatable ring seal. They tape a syringe to it for inflation, to temporize in treating HAPE.

HIGH ALTITUDE COUGH

Although strictly speaking in the absence of HAPE, cough is not an altitude illness. Nevertheless, every group at high altitude usually includes sufferers. Make sure HAPE or a treatable condition such as pneumonia is not present. Cough could be due to asthma, but this appears less likely than at lower altitudes. Facemasks or scarves around the mouth and nose have been proposed to warm the air and increase humidification; however some people taking this approach find it uncomfortable and claustrophobic. Throat lozenges, hard candies, and the like probably help. Keeping a pot of water boiling in a tent to humidify the air has been suggested. Steam inhalations—covering your head and a pot of very hot water with a cloth—and breathing the moist air may help. There is no evidence of benefit from cough suppressants although they could be considered.

TREATMENT PROTOCOLS FOR HEALTH-CARE PROVIDERS AT INTERMEDIATE ALTITUDES

The following protocol is recommended in treating visitors who develop altitude illness on a skiing vacation at intermediate altitudes (9000 feet, 2750 meters). Locations must be modern resorts or towns in developed countries with rapid assured transportation access. Medical people administer the treatment and must be quickly accessible to deal with problems that arise. The scheme is phrased in clinical language, follows the principles of cost containment, and is that used at the clinic in Keystone, Colorado, (9200 feet, 2800 meters) for management of otherwise healthy people without underlying cardiopulmonary conditions.

AMS

If chest is clear on auscultation, then no chest film

- Acetazolamide for sleep
- Oxygen and rest for a severe headache, in addition to aspirin, ibuprofen, or acetaminophen

SUSPECTED HAPE

- Vital signs by a nurse, including temperature (oral). There may be a hypertensive response because of high norepinephrine release with HAPE.

- History and physical by a doctor
- Pulse oximetry on room air (normal at Keystone is 90 to 92 percent, mild cases are between 80 and 90 percent, while readings in the 70s indicate severe HAPE)
- Oxygen by mask or nasal canula (flow rates of 2 to 4 liters per minute as necessary to get oxygen saturation above 90 percent). If the saturation can't be raised to 90 percent with oxygen, then the victim needs to get to a hospital quickly.
- Chest film (may not be needed, but it can sometimes demonstrate unusual conditions, including cardiomegaly or pleural effusion).

Pharmacotherapy of cases
- Nifedipine, 10 mg, bitten and chewed, to see if there is a significant drop in blood pressure and if a clinical response is seen then
- Nifedipine, 20 mg long-acting preparation, twice a day if no clinically significant hypotensive response

Four options for those who wish to optimize a vacation
1. If very sick (especially if confused), then ambulance evacuation to a lower altitude.
2. If moderately sick (hypoxemia not readily corrected with oxygen), then hospitalize overnight, observe, keep on oxygen, monitor, and if better next day, send back to the hotel to rest and keep on oxygen.
3. If less sick (hypoxemia easily corrected with low flow

oxygen), then send back to hotel and have a hospital supply company bring out oxygen to be administered by nasal prongs at 2 liters per minute throughout the night. Check the next day, and if patient recovered to point of being asymptomatic and if chest is clear to auscultation, rest a day and resume normal activity.

4. For very mild cases (just not feeling well, a few rales, small infiltrate on chest film, pulse oximetry above 85 percent), send to hotel room with nifedipine but without oxygen, and recheck the next day.

If no response to nifedipine, then reevaluate and evacuate patient
  - No use of furosemide
  - No CPAP or PEEP, or grunt breathing

HACE

MRI scans are increasingly available, and in a diagnostically confusing situation with diffusion-weighted imaging, the classic findings show increased T2, a signal of the posterior corpus callosum. Clinical recovery may precede MRI improvement. Given the association with HAPE, a chest radiograph makes sense. Rapid recovery is commonly seen if treatment is started at the first sign of HACE.

  - Descent (ambulance evacuation)
  - Oxygen
  - Dexamethasone (8–10 mg initially followed by 4 mg every six hours)

Consider mannitol, other diuretics, and endotracheal intubation with hyperventilation, but such patients can be overventilated, resulting in poor blood flow to the brain.

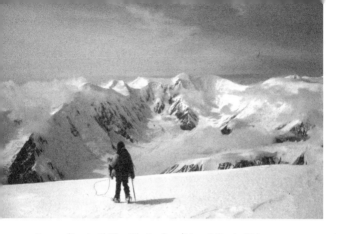

Descending to Chitina Glacier from Mount Steele, Yukon

CHAPTER 6

Going to Altitude with a Preexisting Health Condition

In high altitude environments the relative lack of oxygen has an affect on people, although the dry climate and cold also play a part. For healthy people who acclimatize by ascending slowly, the lack of oxygen is not a problem, at least to intermediate altitudes. Many people go to altitude to exercise, but people with health conditions for which oxygen uptake with exercise at sea level is marginal would be expected to have further difficulties with ascent.

As our population ages, more recognition is given to the beneficial physical, emotional, and psychological effects of exercise. People with financial means are more likely to pay for such experiences, and hence some of these individuals will crave altitude exposure. Older people who travel to altitude for recreation and do so at a reasonable pace may find altitude illness less common. One woman, who died at age 101, regularly climbed Mount Whitney (14,495 feet, 4420 meters) in California up to age 91. However, some may be undertaking an altitude adventure for the first time in their lives, while other seasoned travelers have developed a chronic illness. There are some published reports, but no controlled studies, of lowlanders with chronic diseases going to altitude. Not much is known about the effects of medicines at altitude, and advice by doctors to patients about their medications remains presumptive or speculative and should be taken with caution. In marginal clinical situations where an individual has a strong will and motivation to reach a personal goal, the person might derive a far greater benefit from its possible attainment than from the loss of self-esteem that results from staying at home in a low-risk environment and nursing the chronic illness. I strongly support such efforts providing the sojourner is willing to take risks.

In the period since the first edition of this book appeared, I have received many inquiries from people with various health conditions who want to go to altitude. The general public expects medical science to know far more than it does. So-called evidence-based medicine attempts to specifically isolate questions it studies in order to find effects of various investigations or treatments. The real world is quite different. People have various illnesses and chronic health problems for which there are few specific answers as to what will happen with altitude exposure. As well, certain individuals belong to subgroups with different genetic and socioeconomic status components and will respond differently. Since good studies are lacking, anecdotal reports constitute the bulk of what we know. The material in this chapter may help you make decisions, but recognize its limitations.

If you have a chronic disease such as high blood pressure, a heart condition, or diabetes discuss the proposed altitude journey with your doctor. If she is unfamiliar with the effects of altitude on your disease, refer her to the bibliography at the end of the book. Or look for an expert (see "Websites Related to Altitude Adaption and Illness" in chapter 7). Your doctor working in conjunction with an altitude expert is best. Sound clinical judgment about your health situation, what is known about the effects of altitude, and your sense of risk assumption will guide decision-making.

Some, who should not venture to altitude, may wish to do so despite being advised against it by their doctors and experts. If you fall into the category of having a condition that may be made worse by altitude and you want to go anyway, choose an itinerary with access to easy descent and medical help. Taking along enough oxygen is usually impractical but do bring a hyperbaric bag.

If you have a chronic disease that could cause problems at altitude, attempt an activity near home similar to the one planned. Repeat the same effort at an intermediate altitude (8000 feet, 2440 meters), hopefully near home. If you perform well under both circumstances, consider attempting the activity at higher altitudes. The exercise guidelines described under "Heart Conditions," below, make sense for everyone.

Anyone going to altitude with a group, either commercial or otherwise, should disclose, in appropriate detail, their significant medical conditions to the other members and to the commercial operator before the trip. I may not want to be on a rope with a poorly-controlled seizure patient and would myself have a fit if my epileptic climbing partner didn't disclose this to me beforehand. We owe it to everyone on a trip to be forthcoming with our health problems. Acceptance of someone's health condition is then a group decision, and any difficulties that result will be addressed by everyone.

Advice follows regarding the more common chronic conditions for which altitude exposure can have an effect. Much of this comes from the experience of others, especially Dr. Peter Hackett, whose judgment I continue to admire. Recognize the limitations of the material presented here since careful studies are lacking. If your condition is not listed here, it means that I am unaware of any useful information with this situation at altitude. Please write me (c/o The Mountaineers Books) with your experience afterward.

HIGH BLOOD PRESSURE

Many with hypertension have uneventful journeys to altitude. Individuals with hypertension may find their pressures elevated at altitude because of the increased activity of the sympathetic nervous system. You should eat a low-salt diet and schedule additional rest during the first few days at altitude. Seek advice from a knowledgeable physician regarding your medicines. If your blood pressure is difficult to control, either you or a companion should check it and be prepared to modify your drug regimen. But don't chase your blood pressure readings with drugs. Only consider changes to your medication if the pressure is consistently high or low. Even then, if you're not symptomatic and are staying at altitude for only a brief time, the situation will resolve with descent. Beta blockers (including propranolol, atenolol, and metoprolol), are one category of drugs used to treat high blood pressure, but they're probably not as effective at altitude as they are lower down. People taking these drugs may have less exercise tolerance and more breathlessness at altitude. Clonidine and prazosin may be useful to control pressures at altitude. Other categories of drugs that may be useful at altitude include calcium channel blockers and ACE inhibitors, but there are no controlled studies of any drugs at altitude.

DIABETES

Diabetics on insulin may have significant problems controlling their disease in the mountain environment; however, many do succeed and enjoy the experience. Those on oral medicines are not subject to the same difficulties. Diabetics with retinopathy may have increased risk of the condition progressing at altitude and should have an evaluation of risk by an altitude-savvy eye doctor. Diabetics on insulin who have not traveled to a foreign country or have not undertaken the planned adventure should first take a shakedown trip to get used to monitoring blood sugars and modifying the insulin dose. It is wise to seek careful counseling with a knowledgeable doctor before the trip.

Diabetics may experience problems regulating their insulin dose because of varying energy expenditure and food intake. Absorption of carbohydrates after eating may be delayed by the body, and if insulin is taken before eating, symptomatic hypoglycemia may occur. Taking insulin after dinner may be preferable. More frequent blood glucose determinations and insulin dosing may be necessary. Shorter-acting preparations may make control easier. Insulin needs for diabetic mountaineers at altitude appear to increase even with strenuous exercise. This may plateau or decline with acclimatization.

Some of the self-monitoring glucose devices may not work accurately and read low at altitude. Carry glucagon and a few sugar cubes in case of insulin reactions and instruct companions in their use. Don't let insulin freeze and carry extra in case of loss or breakage. Control the blood sugar so it is in the slightly higher than normal range—but do your best to not let your sugar get too high. Keep hydrated. It may be more difficult to recognize diabetic reactions and to confuse them with AMS. AMS symptoms may lead to not eating enough and require compensating with lower insulin doses to prevent low blood sugar with exercise. At altitude this has resulted in ketoacidosis, the extreme form of deranged sugar control. Diabetics who have let their disease get out of control at altitude have experienced great difficulties in being treated, increasing the risk of death. It is conceivable that taking acetazolamide in such a situation can exacerbate the condition.

NEUROLOGIC CONDITIONS

Transient ischemic attacks (TIAs) and strokes have been reported at high altitude (above 16,000 feet, 4880 meters) in young healthy individuals. Dehydration may be a contributing factor. A TIA is a brief neurologic difficulty, such as one side of the body or an arm or a leg feeling weak or numb. It lasts more than a few minutes, but less than twenty-four hours. If you have such symptoms at altitude, increase hydration, take one aspirin a day, descend immediately, and end the trip. If you have already had a stroke and recovered to function well enough to go to altitude, you can consider going, but we know little about your risks in doing so.

If you have epilepsy and your seizures are controlled on medicines, be sure to continue your drugs at altitude. But if you have recently stopped your anti-seizure medicines at sea level, because you haven't had a seizure in a long time, your seizures may return after abrupt exposure to altitude. Have your doctor consider the drug topiramate for seizure control. Some of its properties are similar to acetazolamide in assisting acclimatization to altitude, although it has not been studied for this purpose.

The slight cerebral edema that develops at altitude may compromise the function of people with brain tumors. Tumors and other central nervous system conditions have first become symptomatic at altitude. Individuals who had a subarachoid aneurysm coiled have successfully gone to intermediate altitudes.

The issue of migraine headaches is dealt in chapter 9.

HEART CONDITIONS

Many people with heart conditions, especially coronary artery disease such as a previous heart attack or coronary bypass surgery, have ventured to altitude successfully and treasure the experience. Heart transplant recipients have climbed Kilimanjaro. In some countries, cardiac rehabilitation programs exist at altitude for sea level dwellers with heart disease. Death while exercising does not appear more common at altitude than at sea level. However those with coronary artery disease who do not exercise at sea level would be ill-advised to begin an exercise regimen at altitude.

What if you have no heart problems but are worried about whether your heart can withstand going to altitude? If you are older than fifty with risk factors for heart disease, you might consult with your doctor who may suggest exercise testing as well other studies if that test were positive. The exercise test, however, can be positive in normal people without heart disease and cause needless worry and expense. Argentinean authorities have been known to require the results of an exercise test on anyone applying to climb Aconcagua.

Heart patients feel a sense of security in North America since they can dial 911 and be rapidly transported to modern emergency departments. In many altitude destinations throughout the world, help can be days away. Keep this in mind as you make your decision to go to such locations.

If you have angina and moderate symptoms, take a number of medicines, and have occasional angina at rest with some exercise limitations, you may tolerate some exposure to altitude. If you have severe angina and limitation of physical effort at sea level, you are probably not reading this book. You should not go to altitude, as lack of oxygen there will increase cardiac work and precipitate severe attacks. If you are going to altitude with angina ascend slowly, increase your anti-anginal medicines, and rest for the first two to three days on arrival. Before your trip talk to your doctor about treating significant blood pressure elevation with prazosin or clonidine. Treat significant anginal symptoms with oxygen if available, and descend without exertion.

If you have had a heart attack (myocardial infarction), coronary bypass surgery, or both, you need not be treated any differently than anyone in the above categories. Get in shape before you go, since the ability to exercise at altitude may be more important than the relative lack of oxygen there. If you don't have a positive exercise study, you may do well. You may have decreased exercise tolerance at altitude and have earlier angina. But you are probably not at a greater risk of having another heart attack at altitude compared to performing the same exercise at sea level.

If you have somewhat controlled congestive heart failure

(CHF) you may get worse at moderate altitude (6500 feet, 1980 meters) or higher. It may be difficult to determine whether your symptoms are due to your congestion getting worse or from mountain sickness. AMS and fluid retention at altitude could aggravate your CHF. If you go to altitude, be prepared to modify your drug regimen and monitor your weight and blood pressure. Consider using acetazolamide prophylaxis.

Individuals with valvular heart disease and complicating pulmonary artery hypertension may be at increased risk of HAPE. Rheumatic heart disease in local people working for you at altitude may predispose them to HAPE. People with a condition called cardiomyopathy may have similar difficulties. The ability to process oxygen at altitude will decline for those with significant valvular disease, and at some point people with limited exercise capacity at sea level will be exhausted performing activities of daily living up high.

Exercise guidelines at altitude are helpful for everyone. Maximal achievable heart rates decline at altitude whether you have heart disease or not. If you have coronary heart disease, having a target heart rate as an end point for activity levels at altitude is better than an activity prescription. From your treadmill test, your doctor can determine 75 percent of the ischemic end-point heart rate at your home altitude. This is your target rate at altitude and would be reasonable for other individuals with chronic disease at altitude. Without an exercise study, you can substitute a derived maximal heart rate (= 206 - 1.2[age - 20]) for the exercise study rate. Watches are available to measure your pulse. Test this rate with strenuous exercise, and see if you can maintain that heart rate comfortably. If not, scale it down to a rate that you can maintain.

LUNG CONDITIONS

Asthma is becoming more common, and deaths from it are increasing. However, many asthmatics report improvement in their condition at altitude, which may be due to less dust, less resistance from a lower air density, and fewer inhaled allergens. In fact there is a sanitarium at 10,500 feet (3200 meters) in Kyrgyzstan devoted to the clinical treatment of asthma! There, asthmatics benefit from taking acetazolamide (250 mg three times a day) before abrupt ascent and for one day afterward. Don't go to altitude before your asthma is stable. If an asthmatic has a severe attack at altitude, it is unknown whether there is an increased risk of death. Asthmatics should be prepared for such situations and carry oral steroids. They should carry their inhaler on a cord around their neck to avoid losing it. Individuals with cold- or exercise-induced asthma may have more attacks at altitude and should use inhaled bronchodilators before exercise as they normally would. An airway warming mask might also be helpful. The use of a spacer for a metered dose inhaler is more important at altitude than at sea level in order to limit evaporation of the medicine in the dry air. Those with exercise-induced asthma should consider using leukotriene inhibitors.

Individuals with mild to moderate chronic lung disease (emphysema or chronic bronchitis) already "live high" because of their compromised lungs. They may tolerate modest altitudes but may be more likely to have AMS and have their health further compromised by altitude. Those on home oxygen should continue this and increase the flow rate by the ratio of the home pressure to the new barometric pressure. Carry a pulse oximeter to monitor your oxygenation. If you have sleep apnea or bad emphysema with marked lowering of oxygen in the arterial blood and retention of carbon dioxide, stay home. If you have sleep apnea, use a CPAP machine at home, and the desire to go anyway, you will need to adjust the machine at altitude if it doesn't have pressure-compensating features. Those with obstructive sleep apnea may do better at altitude than with central forms.

People with pulmonary hypertension from various causes are likely to have difficulties at altitude. Those with congenital heart disease, restrictive lung disease, mitral stenosis, and recurrent pulmonary emboli among others may have increased risk.

GASTROINTESTINAL CONDITIONS

Gastrointestinal bleeding at altitude may be more common than it is at lower altitudes. Certainly there are numerous reports of serious bleeds occurring in climbers. Reasons are speculative. Steroid-induced ulcers from dexamethasone are possible as is use of ibuprofen and other drugs of this class. The situation for people with various preexisting ulcer conditions is unknown. If you do have peptic ulcers, it would be prudent to have your ulcer symptoms under control before going high and to avoid drugs that could provoke bleeding. In case of bleeding, as demonstrated by bloody vomit or stools or dark tarry stools, expeditious descent is advised. Whether or not the acid-reducing drugs would help is unknown, but they should be tried with proton pump inhibitors, such as omeprazole, given priority. Ice water lavage of the stomach was another procedure done in my doctoring youth that might be considered in the cold heights.

BLOOD PROBLEMS

If you have sickle cell disease you should limit altitude exposure and bring oxygen to any significant altitude away from medical facilities. If you have sickle cell trait and other hemoglobin-opathies such as SC, or Hb S, beta+-thalassemia and normal lung function, limit exposure to 10,000 feet (3050 meters) and be aware that your spleen may give you pain. People with some blood abnormalities do not get the rapid breathing and increased pulse at altitude because of improved oxygen loading in the lungs. If you have a spleen (that has not previously become shrunken), breathe supplemental oxygen during air travel (difficult on many airlines) and keep yourself very well hydrated. If you have impaired lung function, problems may occur at altitudes lower than 10,000 feet (3050 meters).

The risk of blood clots is increased at altitudes above 14,000 feet (4270 meters), and possibly lower. Dehydration, increased red blood cells, and not moving while stormbound may increase the risk. Those with a history of blood clotting problems, including deep vein thromboses and pulmonary emboli, are almost certainly at an increased risk in the mountains. Clots may occur in other parts of the body than the lungs and legs. Some expedition doctors carry low-molecular-weight heparin, which could be used to treat suspected clots without the need for laboratory monitoring. The advisability of taking aspirin at altitude to prevent clots is discussed under "Blood Response" in chapter 1.

OBSTETRIC AND GYNECOLOGIC CONDITIONS

While there are no studies demonstrating that birth control pills cause blood clots at altitude, anecdotal reports suggest they are a hazard. Women have been counseled to continue them at least to intermediate altitudes (less than 10,000 feet, 3050 meters), as the risk of pregnancy may be greater than the possible increased risk of blood clots. Short stays at higher altitudes probably pose little hazard. Other experts disagree and advise the use of other contraceptives at altitude.

Women who live at altitude tend to have smaller babies. For pregnant sojourners, there are no studies on which to base advice. Certainly many pregnant women travel to intermediate altitudes for various recreational activities without incident. If you have concerns about the possible adverse effects of altitude on your unborn child, it is best not to go. Some advise against travel to altitude for pregnant women, while others would limit exposure to moderate altitudes (less than 13,125 feet, 4000 meters). Others are concerned that exercise at altitude during pregnancy might compromise fetal oxygenation. A reasonable compromise would be to limit exposure during the first trimester to 8000 feet (2440 meters) for uncomplicated pregnancies, ascend slowly, and not exercise very strenuously. If you have a complicated pregnancy, don't go. If you have had great difficulties conceiving, consider not going. Pregnant women should make every effort to avoid all forms of altitude illness. Any symptom should necessitate expeditious descent. There are no studies in drug treatment of altitude illness in pregnancy.

TAKING CHILDREN TO ALTITUDE

Infants and young children born at sea level may be more at risk from altitude illness than adults, perhaps because recognition of problems by adults may be delayed. If a child is not doing well at altitude it may be more difficult to determine the cause. Existing studies focus mainly on children who reside at altitude; there are no studies of treatments in children who ascend from low altitudes. The Consensus Statement of the International Society for Mountain Medicine (2001) is a helpful guide. Children have been taken to altitudes above 17,000 feet (5180 meters) by responsible adults without incident. I would only advise going to altitude with children if the route permits a flexible itinerary and rapid descent, and only if the child has no underlying conditions, such as congenital heart disease, Down's Syndrome, or epilepsy that might prove problematic at altitude. Colds and upper respiratory illness may increase the risk of altitude illness and may be reasonable grounds for delaying the trip.

Taking very young children to altitude rarely benefits the child, but it can be a memorable family trip if all goes well. School and other organizational trips to altitude present other possibilities, and parents would be wise to make sure the leaders are knowledgeable about altitude and have good judgment.

Try to make the trip as enjoyable for the child as possible. That could be quite difficult if you are not doing well. If it is your first time at altitude don't expose yourself and your child for more than a few hours. Be extremely cautious about sleeping above 2500 to 3000 meters (8200 to 9840 feet) without a gradual ascent. Children should not walk longer than they want to, and a variety of stimulating events and enjoyable food is a must.

See chapter 4 for diagnosing altitude illness in children. The nondrug treatment guidelines suggested make sense for children, with descent involving minimal exertion to be undertaken with any symptoms of suspected altitude illness. Give oxygen if available. There is no documented experience with children in the hyperbaric bag, and I suspect it would be a very scary experience. We do not know about the effectiveness of pharmaceuticals to prevent or treat mountain sickness in children, though some experts would approve using acetazolamide (see chapter 5 for recommended doses). Side effects in children may make it difficult to judge the response. Dexamethasone for treating HACE and nifedipine for HAPE makes sense although descent should always prevail.

MISCELLANEOUS AFFLICTIONS

If your condition has not been mentioned in this book, it appears there is little experience-based information to offer you. A database of travelers to altitude with preexisiting conditions would be helpful. Upon return consider reporting to me what happened to you at altitude.

EYE CONDITIONS

In addition to the retinal bleeds mentioned in chapter 2, people who have had some types of corneal surgery are at risk at altitude. The cornea and retina are very sensitive to oxygen. Depending on age, those who have had radial keratotomy to improve distance vision will have difficulty to the point where they can become nearly blind as they gain altitude. This may occur even below 9840 feet (3000 meters) and can be expected to get worse with increasing age. It usually takes about 24 hours to develop, becoming noticeable the next day. Bring several pairs of eyeglasses of increasing power to correct vision as it is difficult to predict the correction needed. The visual problems do reverse with descent. Young persons may not notice much visual impairment at altitude until they age.

However, people with radial keratotomy have successfully climbed Everest. If you have had this procedure, be sure to inform your companions.

Photorefractive keratectomy done with a laser, another corneal procedure, does not appear to pose such significant problems nor does laser-assisted in-situ keratomileusis (LASIK), which can provide greater improvements in distance vision. However, LASIK may decrease distance vision at altitude to a small degree (like looking through wax paper) in some people at extreme altitudes, but this difficulty may improve with acclimatization. Those with such corneal surgery may suffer from dry eyes at altitude.

Dry eyes affect many people at altitude. In addition to corneal surgery causing problems, certain drugs can diminish tearing and should be avoided up high. Topical tear substitutes and lubricating ointments can be considered, and some ophthalmologists would advise using them prophylactically in individuals subject to dry eyes. Plugging the tear ducts with punctal occluders has been done in some altitude sojourners to lessen dry eye problems. Goggles to protect the eyes from wind and to increase the humidity around the cornea may be helpful. Anyone with only a single functioning eye is advised to use polycarbonate eye protection.

People with glaucoma who are treated with beta-blocking eye drops may become short of breath with altitude or fail to acclimatize. If using such drops at altitude consider pushing the lower eyelid firmly against the nose for one minute after using the medicine. This prevents the eye drops from draining into the nose and being absorbed. Consider other agents, including acetazolamide for treating this condition when going up high. Altitude exposure may injure the optic nerve in people with glaucoma.

CONTACT LENSES

Extended wear contact lenses have been worn to 26,250 feet (8000 meters) without mishap. They carry a tenfold greater risk of infection over daily wear lenses, but many climbers prefer them. Disposable lenses are advised, as there are fewer risks of infection from improper cleaning. The newer hyperoxygen-transmissible, extended-wear soft contacts may be even better. Rigid gas permeable lenses expose the cornea to oxygen but may require more work to care for with daily cleaning. If there is any eye pain or redness while wearing contacts at altitude, remove them. Bring artificial tears and keep them from freezing, and carry eyeglasses. Eye-care materials and solutions are not available in many countries where the highest mountains exist.

DIET PILLS

Some diet pills such as fenfluramine and diethylpropion may increase the risk of getting HAPE, probably because they raise pulmonary artery pressure. Other stimulants may do the same.

ORTHOPEDIC PROBLEMS

Joint problems should not behave any differently at altitude compared to sea level. Bilateral amputees have dragged themselves to lofty summits when their prostheses failed!

CANCER

Cancer in remission or under control is not a reason to avoid altitude. It could even have a beneficial effect on the disease process. However, those who have had radiation to the neck as a treatment may be at greater risk of altitude illness because their carotid bodies that control breathing may not be functioning.

DRUG AND ALTITUDE INTERACTIONS

Very little is known about this subject. I get inquiries from people about whether modifications of doses are needed for psychotropic agents such as lithium, for example. Unfortunately there is little knowledge to guide advice.

INFECTIONS AND HIV/AIDS

The immune system that fights infection may not function well at altitudes above 10,000 feet (3050 meters). People with AMS report more symptoms consistent with infections, such as colds and diarrhea. In some cases of sudden unexplained death at altitude where an autopsy has been done, the findings sometimes suggest a serious infection, such as of the heart, as the cause of death. The HIV-infected traveler to altitude may have more serious problems with infections of the gastrointestinal tract and other organs. Choose a route or itinerary with easy descent as a readily available option since descent to a lower altitude would be the best choice if you suspect any infection.

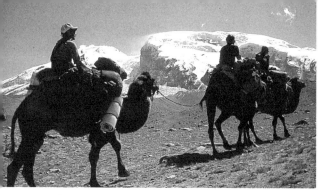
Toward base camp on Muztagh Ata

CHAPTER 7

Preparing to Go to Altitude

You may tolerate the altitude better if you're in good shape to enjoy the activity at altitude. To physically prepare to go to altitude begin by walking in hills with a small daypack. Increase the load, the altitude, and the duration of the exercise. Some athletic women may have low iron stores, making iron supplementation a good idea for them.

If you are mentally prepared for the affair with thin air and have a realistic self-appraisal and a positive attitude, all will likely go well. The mental path depends on your own makeup and what you have done to prepare. Practicing meditation or following other relaxation programs, talking to people with experience in the activity, or seeking religion are effective means of preparation.

ASSEMBLING A HIGH ALTITUDE MEDICAL KIT

Even if you are going on a guided or organized trip to altitude, you should take responsibility for your own health. Some organized trips have sufficient supplies and knowledgeable personnel, but be prepared.

In addition to other medicines in the personal medical kit (see my book *The Pocket Doctor*), I advise anyone going to altitude to carry acetazolamide—even if you are allergic to sulfas, others around you may not be. If you are allergic and are traveling independently, then carry dexamethasone. If you will camp above 12,000 feet (3660 meters—this figure is somewhat arbitrary), then carry nifedipine and dexamethasone as well. If you have had HAPE before, carry nifedipine to any altitude. Consider renting a hyperbaric bag. A pulse oximeter could be useful, although cut-off values for readings at various altitude destinations are unknown, which would hamper decision making. Everything necessary to prevent serious high altitude conditions can be done without the pulse oximeter. Learn about ascent profiles and rescue options, and consider satellite phones or two-way radios for communication.

EVALUATING MODES OF TRAVEL TO ALTITUDE

If traveling to altitude with a commercial group, ask the company staff about the ascent profile and whether oxygen or a hyperbaric bag is carried along? If you are paying for an expensive trip, one or both should be included for sustained trips above 15,000 feet (4570 meters). Inquire about the contents of the medical kit. What is the leader's experience and success in taking clients to altitude? Talk to the leader directly, and ask to talk to clients who have gone to altitude with your leader to get a firsthand opinion of the leader's capabilities. Ask about the altitude experience of other members of the group. Does the company screen its clients or just their wallets? What is the company's experience in trips to high altitude? How often have they had to evacuate people? Have there been any fatalities? Ask to talk to clients who have been on trips where there have been evacuations to form an opinion of the company's safety interests.

What are the options for descent or evacuation on the itinerary? Ask about contingency plans at various points on the ascent profile. For a journey to the Tibetan Plateau, where there are few options for descent, the answer is very important. Determine whether an individual who is not acclimatizing well can leave the group and be escorted down. Don't just take "yes, of course" as an answer; ask for specifics.

If you are going to altitude with friends on a noncommercial basis, create a contingency plan should someone get altitude illness. Decide whether the group wants to take a hyperbaric bag or oxygen and whether there will be communication options for rescue. The ease of descent should altitude illness occur is critical in choice of route.

If you are going with people you don't know well, get a sense of their priorities. Does someone brag, "I'm going to make the summit or die trying"? When he gets in trouble with severe AMS, he may refuse to go down. Or if you get sick, you could be abandoned.

If going solo, consider your route choices for descent, and plan treatment options for altitude illness. What if there is no help nearby?

SPECIFIC SITUATIONS

Common altitude environments and activities warrant discussion here. If you have had AMS, plan to go skiing in one of the mountain states, live near sea level, will stay at a resort town above 6000 feet (1830 meters), and need to ascend quickly, consider taking acetazolamide. For example, if you fly to Denver and plan to go on to Vail, spend the first night in Denver before going higher. Most people do well enough without taking acetazolamide. In one study, more than half the people attending a conference in a hotel at an altitude of 9800 feet (2990 meters) had symptoms of AMS. In another study at altitudes of 6500 feet (1980 meters) a quarter of conference participants had symptoms of mild AMS. Although HAPE is relatively rare, hundreds of cases do occur each year in these places.

If you're flying to Lukla (9200 feet, 2800 meters) in Nepal, a starting point for Everest Base Camp, do not try to get to Namche Bazaar (11,000 feet, 3350 meters) the first day. Follow the ascent guidelines and consider using acetazolamide at night to improve sleep. If you have walked in from Jiri, you will do better. If flying to Lhasa (12,000 feet, 3660 meters) or similar altitudes in South America, consider taking acetazolamide before landing for prevention. If you haven't, use it when you arrive to treat symptoms of AMS and take it easy the first few days.

In climbing a mountain such as Rainier at 14,400 feet (4390 meters) in Washington State, people ascend to 10,000 feet (3050 meters) in one day, camp, and climb to the summit early the next morning. Most people suffer from AMS, although HAPE is almost unheard of unless people get stranded near the top and can't get down. Carry acetazolamide; it could be taken before bedtime to get better sleep. If you want to climb Kilimanjaro, try to arrive in Nairobi (5500 feet, 1680 meters) a few days early to acclimatize. Spend extra days at the higher huts on the ascent. This may be difficult because the guides work against you as they herd people up the mountain. The ascent profile is rapid for most people, so consider taking acetazolamide at night, especially if you have had AMS. If yours is a light alpine style expedition to 19,685 or 22,965 feet (6000 or 7000+ meters), carry acetazolamide, nifedipine, and dexamethasone, but use them only to treat altitude conditions. If you are climbing in the traditional expedition style by establishing a base camp at a high altitude and your route lacks a quick, easy, rapid descent, take a hyperbaric bag and, possibly, oxygen.

Finally, if you are a member of a rescue party that is being flown by helicopter to 17,000 feet (5180 meters) on Mount McKinley (Denali) to find a lost party, take both acetazolamide and dexamethasone before you depart and continue taking them during your stay up high.

THOSE AROUND YOU WHO MAY GET ALTITUDE ILLNESS

It is commonly assumed that people working for altitude adventurers are immune to altitude illness. People who reside at high altitude may be especially prone to reascent HAPE. Lowlanders are just as susceptible as you or even more so, often because of language barriers and by denying symptoms in their desire to earn money. Fatal HACE has been commonly reported among lowland pilgrims to altitude sites. You are responsible for your trip staff and should not assume that staff leaders and bosses have the necessary caring and clinical judgment to make appropriate decisions at altitude. For those on group trips to altitude, consider keeping a daily register of everyone and their symptoms as you travel, as discussed in chapter 9 for leaders. Also be aware of the material on treatment of staff on the International Porter Protection Group website, *www.ippg.net*.

WHERE TO GET MORE INFORMATION

Attend conferences where experts give presentations on altitude illness and ask them questions. The International Hypoxia Symposia (*www.hypoxia.net*) at Lake Louise, Alberta, held in odd years in February is attended by many of the world's experts. The other major conference is sponsored by the International Mountain Medicine Society (*www.ismmed. org*) in various locations in even years. There are several conferences organized on wilderness medicine topics, presented for different types of audiences that include presentations on altitude illness. Speak to doctors at travel medicine clinics to get referrals to those knowledgeable about altitude illness. Pulmonary medicine is one clinical specialty that may have some practitioners understanding the problems at altitude, but family practitioners and those who have worked at altitude providing care to sojourners may be the best source of advice. The journal *High Altitude Medicine and Biology* may be helpful as well as the sources in the bibliography. Talk to others who have been at altitude, ask at local climbing clubs, and talk to people in outdoor equipment stores (the latter being the least reliable option).

WEBSITES RELATED TO ALTITUDE ADAPTATION AND ILLNESS

Search engines will give you plenty of sites with information of variable accuracy and relevance. The experience is comparable to taking a drink from a fire hose. The specific ones listed below may provide a gentler flow of fresh mountain spring water.

International Society of Mountain Medicine. This is the premier group of savvy altitude savants. The website has useful information on altitude conditions and is the best single source of links to related sites. The society may eventually provide a physician referral center for more information. *www.ismmed.org*

International Hypoxia Symposia. This group sponsors the other major meetings on altitude illness. *www.hypoxia.net*

Wilderness Medical Society. This organization addresses a variety of health problems in wilderness settings and provides many useful links. *www.wms.org*

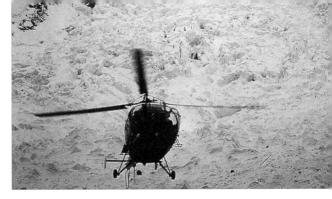

Khumbu Icefall, Mount Everest

CHAPTER 8

Case Studies

Descriptions of people with altitude illness and accounts of how they were treated follow. Complete information is commonly lacking.

SKIER WITH HAPE AT U.S. ALTITUDE DESTINATION WHERE MEDICAL SERVICES ARE READILY AVAILABLE

Reginald, a moderately obese, thirty-year-old salesman from San Francisco, skied occasionally in the Lake Tahoe area. A late snowfall during a March cold spell tempted him to drive to Lake Tahoe (6300 feet, 1920 meters). The next day he skied at Heavenly Valley (between 7000 and 10,000 feet, 2130 and 3050 meters). He then drove to Mammoth Mountain (8000 feet, 2440 meters), where he spent the next two nights, and skied strenuously the next two days between 8000 and 11,000 feet (2440 and 3350 meters). He lost his appetite and did not drink much in the evenings at the bar, as he had done at Tahoe. On the afternoon of the second day at Mammoth, he was very short of breath and weak. He continued to ski though, and by the end of the day he could barely get up the loading ramp to the lift. That night he developed a cough, more shortness of breath, and a noisy chest. Medical help brought him to a hospital where HAPE was diagnosed; he was given nifedipine and kept overnight on oxygen. Feeling normal the next day he returned to his hotel to rest and breathe oxygen obtained from a medical supply company. He was rechecked that evening and was told he could try skiing again if he continued taking nifedipine. He did manage another day of skiing but was not the tiger he thought himself to be.

Analysis: As he tried to be a weekend warrior, Reginald's mild AMS progressed to HAPE. His obesity is a risk factor. He recovered quickly with medical therapy and continued skiing. Victims at altitude resorts in developed countries where there is reliable rapid access to health care can salvage their vacations this way. Such a course would not be advisable on a ski ascent in the Karakorum (Pakistan). Reginald should be cautious about rapid ascents and vigorous activity at altitude in the future. A substantial loss of revenue results from people arriving at altitude resort destinations and not consuming expected quantities of food and beverages due to AMS. The industry is eager to see these vacationers treated for AMS!

CLIMBER IN THE SIERRAS WITH HAPE

Maureen, a twenty-four-year-old student, drove from sea level to a trailhead in the Sierra Nevada and slept at 8000 feet

(2440 meters). She was attempting to climb a 14,000-foot (4270-meter) peak over a long weekend. Maureen had slept at altitudes greater than 10,825 feet (3300 meters) on several similar climbing trips and had experienced mild AMS on half of those. She was in good physical shape, running 20 miles a week. She awoke with a headache and slight dizziness, but she didn't tell her male companions and continued with them to 10,500 feet (3200 meters). Her headache improved with aspirin, but she slept fitfully. While climbing the following afternoon, she felt weak, became extremely short of breath ascending, and held the party back. Her headache got worse, and they bivouacked that night at 12,000 feet (3660 meters) without reaching the summit. She stated that her chest felt raspy, and she sensed gurgling there. In addition, she had a dry cough and couldn't sleep. The morning of her third day, Maureen's cough and headache were much worse, and she became very weak and had extreme difficulty breathing. She was helped down to 9025 feet (2750 meters), while one of her partners headed out to get an air rescue. Maureen improved slightly that night. The next morning she was evacuated by helicopter to a hospital at 4200 feet (1280 meters). She was found to have X-ray changes typical of HAPE and she recovered with oxygen.

Analysis: Easy, rapid access to high altitude is improving all over the world. Maureen's physical conditioning and goal orientation for this weekend climb allowed her to ascend rapidly. She denied the worsening symptoms of ascent. When she lost her ability to keep up with them, her companions should have got her down instead of bivouacking at altitude. Rapid ascents are best avoided in the future, and she should consider using nifedipine for prophylaxis if it recurs on further climbs.

MCKINLEY CLIMBER WITH HACE

Kim, a thirty-four-year-old computer programmer from Korea, came to climb Denali (20,320 feet, 6194 meters) solo. He had previously climbed in the Alps. Kim ascended from the airstrip (7300 feet, 2225 meters) and less than two days later, made camp at 14,000 feet (4270 meters) in a snow cave on the West Buttress route. The next day he was found by other climbers, stumbling and confused, but still attempting to ascend. They abandoned their ascent, gave him dexamethasone, acetazolamide, and nifedipine, and took turns carrying and dragging him down. He did not improve much as they struggled to get him to 10,000 feet (3050 meters). However, they were able to complete the evacuation to the "airport" and by then his symptoms had cleared. He couldn't remember what had happened and wanted to continue his ascent, but his rescuers' opinions prevailed and he was flown out.

Analysis: The ascent rate in this highly motivated climber was far too rapid. He developed HACE and was lucky that climbers were nearby and willing to help. Their treatment was shotgun, as is often the case in desperate situations. Getting an ataxic climber down on a big mountain is challenging. Sometimes cooking in a snow cave or snow-covered tent has produced carbon monoxide intoxication that presents with similar symptoms.

TREKKER TO MOUNT EVEREST FROM THE NORTH WITH FATAL HAPE

Robert, a forty-one-year-old engineer, was a member of "The Highest Trek in the World," whose destination was Camp 3 (20,800 feet, 6340 meters) on Everest. He had previously climbed Kilimanjaro (19,340 feet, 5895 meters) and wanted to get above 6000 meters (19,685 feet). Because of a delayed business deal, he flew to Lhasa (12,000 feet, 3660 meters) two days behind his trekking party. After two nights in Lhasa, Robert hired a jeep to catch up with the group. He avoided medicines on religious grounds and did not take any acetazolamide. He was driven to the Everest Base Camp (16,900 feet, 5150 meters) in three days. Upon arrival at the base camp, he was found to have a severe headache and nausea. The jeep departed. Against his wishes, he was given 500 mg of acetazolamide, but the next morning the symptoms continued and he vomited several times. The trip leader felt the vomiting was due to the large dose of acetazolamide and gave him another medicine for vomiting. He suggested Robert descend on a yak, but Robert refused, saying he would be fine after a night's sleep. That night he had a nonproductive cough for which he was given some cough medicine. He awoke with extreme shortness of breath and was diagnosed with HAPE. Another party at base camp that was preparing to descend had a Gamow Bag, and Robert was put into it for a total of 3 hours. After the first 2 hours, he asked to come out of the bag and quickly became breathless again. He spent another hour inside and came out of the bag feeling much better. The other party descended with the bag. Robert felt too sick to continue up to Camp 3 but said he would improve at base camp. His party proceeded with their scheduled itinerary, leaving later that day while an attendant remained with him. That night he slept in the tent by himself, and in the morning he was found dead.

Analysis: The tendency for reckless rapid ascent profiles is common at many locations including Tibet. Hurried vacations, demanding itineraries, and the difficulties in arranging quick rescue are hazards of travel today. This case illustrates some of the realities of commercial trips. In an attempt to achieve his goal, Robert ascended far too quickly. Once severe AMS was diagnosed, descent options were limited, and in an attempt to please the client, the leader did not require him to go down and apparently abandoned his supervisory role. The victim of altitude illness is rarely competent to make decisions about his care. Continued access to the Gamow Bag was also problematic. Descent should have been undertaken by yak or porter, and he should not have been allowed to sleep in the tent alone.

TREKKER DOCTOR TO MOUNT EVEREST IN NEPAL DYING OF HAPE

George, a sixty-two-year-old doctor, had been evacuated from Mount Kenya (17,058 feet, 5199 meters) in February with HAPE that improved immediately on descent. In the spring he walked from Jiri (6250 feet, 1905 meters) to Gorak Shep (17,000 feet, 5180 meters) in Nepal's Everest region over the course of ten days. He developed a dry cough, and his medical companion gave him a furosemide injection while attempting descent. An air rescue was launched and three days later he ended up in a Kathmandu hospital, where he continued to be short of breath and blue in spite of oxygen treatment. He deteriorated and died 26 hours after admission, despite heroic attempts to treat him.

Analysis: There was no attempt to prevent HAPE by taking nifedipine, the ascent rate was too fast, descent was delayed waiting for an air evacuation, and the medical treatment in the field was inappropriate. Although he descended to a lower altitude, he deteriorated probably because the initial HAPE process, which was a lung injury, had progressed to irreversible lung disease as confirmed by autopsy. In the only study of autopsy findings on trekkers dying of altitude illness in Nepal, three out of seven were physicians!

TREKKER TO MOUNT EVEREST IN NEPAL DYING OF SEVERE AMS

John, a fit and experienced forty-one-year-old, trekked with his wife and friends to reach Kala Pattar. He had experienced some dizzy spells at lower altitudes, but the spells had occurred occasionally throughout his life without problems. After a rest day at Namche (11,000 feet, 3350 meters), they ascended to Tengboche (12,887 feet, 3876 meters), where John noted a headache the next morning. They continued to Pheriche (13,950 feet, 4252 meters) to spend the night and walked up the side valley the next day, returning to Pheriche to sleep. John's headache persisted, and his appetite was OK. He visited the Himalayan Rescue Association's aid post doctor but didn't disclose that he had a headache. The next morning he continued up to Lobuje (16,175 feet, 4930 meters) with difficulty maintaining his balance, which he passed off to his dizziness, but he remained in good spirits. After spending the night in Lobuje, the group set out for Kala Pattar (18,450 feet, 5623 meters), but John was too weak to make it to the foot of the ascent and was helped back to Lobuje, arriving at 4:30 in the afternoon. Because it was late in the day they decided to have him rest overnight and descend the next day. John went straight to bed, having no interest in dinner. At 7:30 P.M. he was checked on and could answer questions. At 1:30 A.M. his wife could not awaken him. He was comatose, unresponsive, and in the next twenty minutes his heart stopped. CPR was performed for two hours without success.

Analysis: This was not an unreasonable ascent profile, but ascent with a headache to sleep at a higher altitude turned out to be fatal. John did not mention his symptoms to the HRA doctor, who would have told him not to ascend the next day. His good spirits masked his underlying progression to severe AMS. Attempted exercise the next day with severe weakness led to a late return, and the group decided tragically to wait until morning to descend. With symptom deterioration it is never too late to descend, and it is possible that if he had been carried down to Pheriche that evening, he might have lived. This case demonstrates the danger of passing symptoms off on another condition, not divulging symptoms, and companions being distracted by the victim's good spirits.

TREKKER CHILDREN WITH ALTITUDE ILLNESS IN NEPAL

Adina, six years old, traveled to Everest Base Camp from Jiri (6250 feet, 1905 meters) with her nine-year-old brother and mother and father. They had a slow pace, with Adina walking or being carried. She was energetic and cheerful and was noted to walk well from Dingboche (14,250 feet, 4340 meters) to Lobuje (16,175 feet, 4930 meters). The next day she arrived at Gorak Shep (17,000 feet, 5180 meters) and by nightfall was in the tent. After dinner she complained to her parents that she felt she wasn't able to "walk quite right." They had not noticed anything unusual up to this point. Testing tandem walking in the tent they found she had balance problems. The parents discussed this with their Sherpa Sardar, who said they had to take her down immediately. Preparations were made to take her down to Lobuje in the dark. As they were leaving the trek leader expressed displeasure at not being consulted, despite the parents previous discussions with him about descending should there be any questions about the children. Her father, carrying her with the Sardar, followed the porter, and by the time she got down to Lobuje, she stopped complaining and was fine. Adina played happily the next day, making mud pies with a local child whose mother was doing the laundry in a nearby stream. The trek leader subsequently complained to the parents about insubordination and endangering the Sherpas who had to cross the glacier at night. He felt Adina should have been allowed to sleep at Gorak Shep and if the parents were concerned they could rouse her from sleep. Recriminations continued for the remainder of the trek as they walked back to Jiri.

Michael, four months old, was taken by his parents to the Annapurna Sanctuary and arrived at the Machhapuchhre Base Camp (12,150 feet, 3700 meters) during a gradual ascent. They were new parents but had trekked considerably before. However, it was a different situation with an infant. On arrival he didn't seem to be his usual somewhat-cranky self. By morning, he was no better, and rather than go up, they descended and his demeanor improved dramatically.

Analysis: At altitude it may be difficult for parents to notice what is happening to their children, as they may be having their own concerns with the altitude. In Adina's case, as soon as she complained, her parents noticed ataxia and called attention to this with the Sherpa Sardar, who decided to descend with her in the dark, which is routine for people who live in this region. Even if such people weren't available to carry her down, it would be prudent not to wait until morning. Rousing a young child from sleep in the middle of the night to check mental status would be problematic as many children do not wake easily from a sound sleep.

Michael's parents took a little time to recognize that his behavior was abnormal, which is probably not unusual for first-time parents who had not previously traveled at altitude with their infant. Descent that evening would have been preferable.

TREKKER TO MOUNT EVEREST IN NEPAL WHOSE HEADACHE CAME ON DURING DESCENT

Alfred was a fit seventy-two-year-old man who wanted to savor the heights yet again and took his time ascending slowly with companions who looked out for one another. He flew to Lukla (9200 feet, 2800 meters) and with proper acclimatization, walked to Lobuje. In what he called the best day of his life, he reached Kala Pattar (18,450 feet, 5620 meters) and then returned to sleep at Lobuje (16,175 feet, 4930 meters). Feeling on top of the world, he sauntered down to Pheriche (13,950 feet, 4250 meters) the next day with no complaints. He went to sleep but woke up at night with a severe headache and nausea. After taking some acetaminophen for pain he went back to sleep, but an hour later he was found unconscious. HACE was suspected, and he was put in the hyperbaric bag, where he improved dramatically. However, HACE didn't necessarily make sense because his symptoms came on with descent, so the next day after descending on foot to 12,795 feet (3900 meters) he was evacuated by helicopter to Kathmandu. Upon arrival he had a normal exam but complained of neck pain. An MRI scan was done and was normal. A week later in Kathmandu, he suddenly became confused and vomited. As part of his further medical workup, a spinal tap was performed, and the fluid demonstrated signs that he had had a bleed in his brain. This subarachnoid bleed (bleeding from a leaking artery in the brain), which was considered a possibility by the doctors at Pheriche, was determined to be the original cause of his symptoms. He eventually had a study demonstrating a cerebral aneurysm, and his artery was clipped. He looks forward to many more years.

Analysis: Be wary of symptoms that come on with descent and yet are diagnosed as altitude illness. HACE does not present with a sudden loss of consciousness, but there is usually a gradual progression of symptoms. Even though there may be a response to treatment, this case demonstrates how there can be another finding which requires attention. This case also represents how difficult it may be to determine the actual cause at altitude. Maintain a high level of suspicion for other causes especially when the clinical presentation is atypical. Similar diagnostic confusion occurs at sea level as well.

HIMALAYAN CLIMBER WITH AMS AND HAPE

Albert, a thirty-two-year-old teacher, flew from Kathmandu to Lukla (9200 feet, 2800 meters) and took 500 mg of acetazolamide daily to prevent AMS. He took three days to ascend to a base camp of 17,700 feet (5390 meters) and arrived with a significant headache and loss of appetite. He joined two friends who had climbed a trekking peak in the Khumbu to undertake a demanding alpine ascent. In two days they reached 22,640 feet (6900 meters), where they camped. During the night Albert developed shortness of breath and a rapidly worsening cough. In the morning he was extremely short of breath, coughing, and almost unable to get out of the tent. His companions recognized that he had HAPE and gave him 10 mg of nifedipine. In fifteen minutes Albert felt his breathlessness was slightly better, and he coughed less. He was soon able to slowly ascend 300 feet (100 meters) and traverse to an easier descent route. There he took 20 mg of the slow-release preparation of nifedipine and descended to the 22,640-foot (6900-meter) camp on his own. That night he had another episode of HAPE that he treated with 20 mg of nifedipine under the tongue, followed by 20 mg of the slow-release preparation. He was able to descend to 16,400 feet (5000 meters) the next day and had no further respiratory problems. He did not resume his climb.

Analysis: This case demonstrates that taking acetazolamide neither prevents HAPE nor masks the symptoms of it. Flights to altitude are always more risky than gradual ascents. The dose of acetazolamide was probably higher than necessary. Acetazolamide does not guarantee that you won't get AMS, especially when ascending rapidly, it just lessens the chances. After ascending too quickly, he joined friends who were already acclimatized. Climbing alpine style presents risks especially to climbers who don't take enough time for acclimatization. Albert did not rest or do short day climbs when he had symptoms of AMS. His continued ascent profile was too rapid. HAPE was treated in the field with nifedipine. He should not have descended alone. Besides a more gradual ascent in the future, if HAPE occurs under such circumstances Albert should consider taking nifedipine for prophylaxis.

KILIMANJARO CLIMBER WITH SEVERE AMS

Gail, a forty-year-old nurse in good physical condition, had climbed to the summit of Mount Whitney (14,495 feet, 4420 meters) three months before she went to Kilimanjaro. Her group followed a standard strategy for the climb of Kili, Africa's highest peak at 19,340 feet (5890 meters). After spending the night in Marangu at 4920 feet (1500 meters), a subtropical oasis, they hiked to Mandara Hut (8860 feet, 2,700 meters), rested, and spent the night. They went on to Horombo Hut (12,200 feet, 3720 meters), where they spent two nights before continuing up to Kibo Hut at 15,420 feet (4700 meters). Gail kept up a good pace throughout. She felt fine and did not take acetazolamide, although other members of her group did. Reaching Kibo, she felt some shortness of breath and slowed her pace but did not become seriously ill. On the attempt to reach the summit the next morning, Gail started out strong but fell behind after 2 hours. She was ataxic, had difficulty breathing, and had to stop to rest after every step in spite of supreme effort to keep going. Her condition deteriorated rapidly. She began to vomit and was forced to turn back several hundred feet short of Gilman's Point on the edge of the crater. Gail descended to Kibo Hut with her guide's assistance and then on to Horombo. Within a couple of hours, she felt fine again.

Analysis: Gail had attempted to preacclimatize on Mount Whitney, but there is little residual effect after three months. A week's stay in Leadville, Colorado (10,170 feet, 3100 meters), just prior to departure may have been preferable. She most likely had mild HACE, which usually clears rapidly with descent. HAPE can take much longer to resolve, especially if it has been present for some time. Many people get altitude illness as they are rushed up Kilimanjaro by guides. It is wise to do all you can to slow the ascent rate.

CLIMBING ACONCAGUA AFTER CARDIAC BYPASS SURGERY

Harry, an experienced fifty-one-year-old climber and lawyer, underwent coronary artery bypass surgery a year ago after a heart attack. He had recovered fully, was symptom free, exercising regularly, and climbing peaks near home. He wanted to fulfill his dream of climbing Aconcagua, the highest summit in the Americas (22,834 feet, 6960 meters).

His doctor advised him against it, and he subsequently was diagnosed with clinical depression. He sought out advice at a meeting of altitude researchers. A lively debate ensued, and he realized there was no strong consensus among the experts. He accepted the risk of being far from help should problems arise, joined a commercial climb that included a climbing doctor, and informed the others on the expedition of his condition. A treadmill test was done as required by the Argentinean authorities. He prepared by exercising in Colorado around 10,000 feet (3050 meters) for a week before departure and perfected pacing himself with his target heart rate. During the trip to base camp he took acetazolamide and monitored his blood pressure. He avoided strenuous carries for the first few days, and then began humping moderate loads and watched his pace by monitoring his pulse. He experienced no unexpected problems. Bad weather prevented them from reaching the summit, but he did reach the team's high point of 20,000 feet (6095 meters) without incident. Upon arrival back home, his mood remained good. Although he has no desire to return to Aconcagua, he continues moderate climbs.

Analysis: A reasoning person may accept risks and behave in a responsible manner toward his climbing companions. Some trekkers and climbers have not told their partners on a venture about their chronic illness and then deteriorated up high and imposed an unexpected burden on the others.

SEVERE FATIGUE AND LASSITUDE AT HIGH ALTITUDE

A forty-two-year-old climber with a history of HACE attempted to climb a trekking peak in Nepal, ascended slowly, and took acetazolamide prophylaxis. He moved to the high camp at 18,965 feet (5780 meters) much slower than the others in his party. The next day he fell behind considerably with no signs of HAPE or HACE. He didn't complain of a headache, but he felt he didn't have enough energy to continue and descended very slowly, resting often. Back at camp he required frequent encouragement to eat and drink. The next four days of travel between 15,750 and 18,375 feet (4800 and 5600 meters) he was very slow and required more prodding to eat and take care of himself. He took a two-day course of nifedipine with no change in fatigue. Within two days of descending to 9850 feet (3000 meters) he regained his former strength.

Analysis: This case was presented to experts on altitude illness in the journal *High Altitude Medicine and Biology* for their opinion on whether his problem was altitude illness, despite having no signs or symptoms except lassitude. One expert suggested he was not supplying enough oxygen to his brain, something called high altitude deterioration, found more commonly above 22,965 feet (7000 meters). He could have had mild AMS without a headache. There was also speculation about an underlying illness that was unmasked by altitude. Psychiatric depression is reported by some to be more common at altitude and could account for the findings. Other experts described situations in which they had seen similar lassitude accompanied by shortness of breath without explanation that slowly resolved itself. Perhaps he just had a few off days or acute mountain lassitude (AML). That is OK.

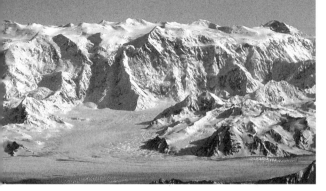

North Face, Mount Logan from Lucania

CHAPTER 9

Questions and Answers

Some people find they learn better by reading answers to questions than by reading plain text.

GENERAL ISSUES ABOUT ALTITUDE

1. I've never been to altitude before. What should I worry about in going there?

Nothing! Going to altitude is a pleasurable experience providing you don't ascend too quickly. Do pay attention to changes in your functioning; monitor how tired you are and your recovery time from an activity. If you're not doing so well, don't raise your sleeping altitude until you are feeling better. If this doesn't work, go down to the altitude at which you first noticed any symptoms of altitude illness.

2. Is good physical fitness protective for altitude illness?

No. Individuals may experience more altitude illness because they can go higher more quickly. Fit people find it easier to enjoy activities at altitude. They should not try to compete with high altitude natives such as Sherpas, who are in their element.

3. What is a good pace at altitude?

One that does not exhaust you and allows you to walk all day without extreme fatigue. A common beginner mistake is to walk too quickly and make frequent rest stops. Follow a rate of activity that does not require you to rest every fifteen minutes or half an hour. Learn the rest step for climbing: Advance your foot, and after placing it on the hill, before bearing weight on it, rest briefly. Then shift your weight and repeat. Synchronize your breathing with your climbing. Whether you're low down on steep ascents or higher, inhale on one step and exhale on the next. At extreme altitudes, take two or three breaths with every step at a rhythm that you can continue without stopping to rest. Repeat a verse of a song or a mantra in synchrony with your feet and lungs. Vary the pace depending on the trail and conditions of the climb. Speed up on easier sections, slow down on more strenuous. Begin the day's journey slowly, and as the muscles and cardiovascular system have "stretched," increase the pace. Toward the end of the day, slow down as the machine is more fatigued.

The other less common mistake people make is to walk too slowly, which is fatiguing in itself. Walk at your pace and not that of the person in front of you. A certain level of discomfort in exercising at altitude (and at sea level) must be tolerated.

4. What is the safe daily rate of ascent at altitude?

No rate is safe for all. Published itineraries for groups going to high altitude on commercial or private trips will be too fast for perhaps 10 to 20 percent of the participants. Not raising the sleeping altitude more than 1000 feet (300 meters) a day above 10,000 feet (3050 meters) is offered as a safe rate of ascent if a stopover day is thrown in every 2000 or 3000 feet (610 or 910 meters). On the stopover day climb as high as you like but return to the previous night's altitude to sleep. Some people will find this too fast, so if they get AMS, they should slow down.

5. If I have altitude illness, does that mean that I will never be a successful high altitude climber?

No. It is OK to have altitude illness. Many Everest summiters have had HAPE and HACE. It is not OK to die from altitude illness, which is a totally preventable condition that if diagnosed and treated early enough results in complete recovery.

6. I had HAPE at 14,000 feet (4270 meters). Does that mean I will always get it at this altitude?

No, it varies with each excursion to altitude. If you ascend slow enough, you will not get it.

7. I've tried to climb Mount Rainier numerous times and find that I always can't go higher than 12,000 feet (3660 meters). Is there a ceiling for certain individuals at altitude?

Perhaps. Try acetazolamide before and during the ascent, and spend an extra day or two at the lower camp before attempting the summit.

8. Are men more likely to get altitude illness than women?

More victims are male, but more men go to altitude. Women tend to breathe more at altitude than men suggesting they may be less susceptible to HAPE. Menstruation in women is probably not a risk factor for getting altitude illness. Also they are less macho and more silent and goal oriented. Men and women are equally at risk.

9. Should I take birth control pills at altitude?

Yes, if you need them for contraception or menstrual regulation to prevent excess bleeding. There is no evidence that it is harmful to take them at altitude, although on theoretical grounds, estrogen-containing oral contraceptives may increase the risk of blood clots higher. Certain individuals with a history of blood clots or a family history of clotting problems (i.e., having a susceptible genetic makeup) may be at an increased risk for blood clot complications. These are more likely to show up in the first year of oral contraceptive use. So beginning the estrogen-containing drugs with no previous history of use and going to altitude soon after is probably risky.

10. Is consuming alcohol bad for acclimatization at altitude?

Probably. The early symptoms of altitude illness resemble those of a hangover. By imbibing, it may be difficult to tell whether you are suffering from altitude illness or from the effects of alcohol. Alcohol depresses respiration during sleep. Avoid alcohol until you are well acclimatized and not going higher.

11. Can judgment be impaired at altitude?

Yes. Psychometric studies on individuals at high altitude show a loss of performance.

12. I'm going to altitude with a commercial group that is carrying a hyperbaric bag. Doesn't that lessen my chances of having problems with serious altitude illness?

No. It is unclear whether a group carrying a hyperbaric bag is less likely to have problems. Among trekkers to high altitude destinations in Nepal, those traveling independently are less likely to experience a fatality resulting from altitude illness. Such people may be more flexible in their schedules and less likely to be influenced by peer pressure. The bag may not change that (see Shlim and Gallie 1992). Aggregate statistics do not distinguish between groups with experienced, competent leaders and those without. Travelers with commercial groups should assess the competence of their leaders as there are no regulatory standards.

13. I feel myself suffocating and not sleeping well at altitude. I catch myself falling asleep and suddenly waking up and feeling claustrophobic in the tent. What should I do?

Avoid sleeping pills and take acetazolamide at bedtime.

14. I live at sea level. Are my chances of getting AMS greater than someone who lives at 5000 feet (1525 meters) or higher?

Yes.

15. What is the finger test for altitude?

The finger test is a term referred to in measuring the oxygen saturation of the arterial blood using a device called a pulse oximeter in which a sensor is attached to the end of a finger. The reading represents the percentage of hemoglobin that is saturated with oxygen in the arterial blood. As one climbs higher, less oxygen is available to fill the oxygen-binding sites on the hemoglobin molecule. There is an expected range for oxygen saturation in the normal individual at particular altitudes and in the person that is acclimatized to that altitude. Newcomers will have lower readings that will increase after a stay at that altitude. Individuals with HAPE will have lower readings. At sea level the normal reading is 96 percent or above, while at 15,000 feet (4570 meters) it is around 86 percent, dropping to about 76 percent around 20,000 feet (6100 meters). At the summit of Everest 29,029 feet (8850 meters) it drops to approximately 58 percent.

Some groups at altitude carry a pulse oximeter (today's models are small and light in weight) in an attempt to gauge how well individuals are acclimatizing and hoping to diagnose HAPE if necessary. Cold fingers as well as exercise can give falsely low readings. And readings may be normal with carbon monoxide poisoning. I feel carrying such a device is unnecessary, but in these technological times, a number of groups do.

16. Up high I lose all my sexual drive. Is this normal?

Yes, although others report an increased libido, an erotic hypoxia.

PHARMACOLOGIC PREVENTION AND THERAPY OF ALTITUDE ILLNESS

1. I'm going to altitude. Should I take acetazolamide to prevent altitude illness?

No, unless you have predictably and repeatedly had altitude illness before and are contemplating another venture up high, or if you are on specific time-cramped itineraries or flying to high-altitude destinations such as Lhasa, Tibet. Use of this agent in our pharmaceutical culture is becoming more common. One individual said, "I feel totally diamoxalized" on a 5000-meter pass. Consider whether this is how you want to remember your affair with thin air.

2. At what altitude should I start to take acetazolamide for preventing altitude illness, given that I have decided to take it?

Just before any abrupt increase in altitude above 8000 feet (2450 meters) beginning the day you ascend.

3. What dosage of acetazolamide should I take when using it for prevention?

Take 125 mg (half a tablet) twice a day, morning and night, if you are ascending slowly to modest altitudes. On the other hand, if you are being transported to significant altitudes, double the dose.

4. Can taking acetazolamide mask the symptoms of altitude illness?

No.

5. I'm allergic to sulfa drugs. Should I take any other drug for preventing altitude illness?

See chapter 3.

6. Will I get rebound altitude illness if I stop taking acetazolamide?

No. It actually aids acclimatization. Stopping dexamethasone, the other prophylactic, can result in rebound.

7. I read the package insert on acetazolamide. So many side effects are listed. Which ones are commonly reported at altitude?

Every side effect ever reported is listed in the manufacturer's statement. Tingling of the lips, fingers, and toes is common as well as urinating more often. While it changes the taste of carbonated beverages, many people don't report this. On rare occasions people do have serious reactions.

8. Acetazolamide, by your accounts, is a great drug. Why not recommend everyone take it at altitude?

I believe in avoiding drugs if there are equally effective and potentially safer alternatives such as slow ascent for altitude. If you believe in a pill for every ill, you may want to act differently. Many people find the tingling that it causes annoying.

9. My doctor suggested I take a sleeping pill since restful sleep is said to be hard to come by at altitude. Is there anything wrong with that?

Yes. Sleeping pills were routinely prescribed by doctors a few decades ago to ensure a good sleep at altitude. Because they depress respiration, a critical factor in acclimatization, taking sleeping pills, sedatives, or tranquilizers is generally not recommended. That said, there are some studies on agents such as temazepam that imply that they do not depress respiration at altitude. Temazepam stays in the blood a long time, and could have an effect on energy levels and motivation. On a climb to 7500 meters that I participated in, two individuals who took a similar drug at altitude were very sluggish the next day, and one climber did not have enough drive to get to the summit. Very short-acting agents have not been studied, but they might also be effective.

10. Now that there is a drug to treat HAPE, isn't altitude illness a less serious problem?

No. Nifedipine has received attention because of its reported ability to help symptoms of HAPE. It has proven very useful in preventing HAPE on rapid ascents of Monta Rosa in the Alps and in studies done by Oswald Oelz and Peter Bärtsch, among others. The treatment effect does not appear to be as dramatic in HAPE that comes on during slower ascents in the Himalaya. People have died, presumably from HAPE, after taking nifedipine.

11. Aspirin has been touted as panacea for extending life and preventing heart attacks. Should I take it at altitude?

Maybe. If you take it on a regular basis at home, then continue taking it at altitude. Whether or not aspirin really is beneficial in sojourners to altitude is unknown. There are theoretical grounds for taking it, at least at extreme altitude (above 18,000 feet, 5590 meters), but it doesn't make sense for everyone at altitudes below that. Discuss this with an altitude-savvy doctor.

12. What about taking furosemide and other potent diuretics at altitude?

Don't. Initial studies supported their use in preventing altitude illness, but they have not been repeated successfully to justify using them at present. Significant side effects, including dehydration and fainting, result from their use. Faced with a serious case of HAPE, most clinicians who carry the drug will likely administer it.

13. Do antacids prevent altitude illness?

No. Experiments conducted to test the hypothesis did not show any effect.

14. My friends are trying to get me to take dexamethasone whenever we climb above 14,000 feet (4270 meters). They say it makes them feel great and perform better. What do you think?

Some people feel dexamethasone, a steroid, is a wonder drug. The controlled, double-blind studies did not show it to be so wonderful. It does prevent AMS but does not aid acclimatization, as acetazolamide does. Acetazolamide both prevents and treats AMS. Steroids can cause euphoria or depression. In addition, if your pills were to get lost or avalanched off, you would be in dire straits. The side effect profile does not warrant even thinking of using this drug routinely. Competitive athletes are disqualified for using this pharmacologic agent; should climbers be any different?

15. In early expedition accounts, climbers carried amphetamines and other stimulants to help when something bad happened or when they were extremely exhausted. Is this a good idea?

The above points about "doping" with steroids apply here. Use of stimulants is hazardous, especially in critical situations requiring good judgment. Studies at low altitudes demonstrate users having poor judgment and being more likely to have a serious automobile accident. Amphetamines have caused death through a variety of mechanisms and produce tunnel vision, which can be hazardous in mountain environments. Modafinil, which has been touted as a modern drug to ward off sleepiness, appears to be difficult to self-monitor (how well you perform) after sleep deprivation. These agents might increase pulmonary artery pressure and lead to HAPE, but there are no studies of any such agents at altitude. The so-called Triple D (dexamethasone, dextroamphetamine, and Diamox) is used by some climbers, just as heroin used to be taken by famous surgeons. I used to carry dextroamphetamine in my medical kit years ago and never used it. Now I don't carry it at all. Use of such agents has been presumed to be the cause of death in some climbers when it affected their judgment, causing them to do something stupid. One climber described having to consciously prevent himself from flying off the mountain while on amphetamines. My sense is that there is considerable use of these agents and likely considerable harm, including death as a result. I speculate that if climbing at altitude was safe, there would be a different population who did the activity. Adding other potential risks may not matter that much for some.

DIET AND HYDRATION RELATED TO ALTITUDE ILLNESS

1. Is there a special diet that is to be recommended at altitude?

While on theoretical grounds, a low fat, high carbohydrate, low salt diet could be best, there are few dietary options for those visiting high altitudes and eating locally produced foods, which usually include meat and potatoes. Eating very salty foods has been reported to increase the risk of altitude illness. A good appetite is a sign of adaptive acclimatization at altitude but can't be relied upon to exclude altitude illness. Eat what appeals to you and is easy to prepare. The widely touted high-energy foods may not be palatable up high and thus not get eaten. Thin people welcome some fat in the diet to help keep insulation from melting away. Garlic may be beneficial.

2. Will keeping well hydrated prevent altitude illness?
Hydration by itself will probably not prevent altitude illness. One can easily get dehydrated at high altitude because the ambient air is so dry, and activity increases insensitive loss. Dehydration may increase the risk of developing altitude illness. Drinking enough water requires effort at altitude—melting snow or purifying a liquid source—but trip leaders report that keeping well hydrated is an important factor for success. In some parts of the world people are advised not to drink water during the day's activities but to hydrate before and after. The timing of hydration has not been adequately studied, but I advise frequent hydration. Like any advice, it can be overdone and people have died from drinking too much water.

Soup mixes, drink powders, instant eggnog, cider, cocoa, and herbal teas make water more palatable and easier to consume in quantity at altitude.

3. All this talk about hydration when the syndromes

to be feared most are excess water in the brain and the lungs. Shouldn't we be drinking less?

No. The waterlogging of the brain or lungs is not a problem of water overload but of leakage from spaces where water is to spaces where it shouldn't be. The lack of oxygen in cells causes this, not an excess of water.

4. *I'm incredibly thirsty at high camp, but I lost my water purification materials. Can I drink the water here anyway?*

Yes. Treating significant dehydration when it occurs takes precedence over the cleanliness of the water source. Melted snow is safe enough as are mountain water sources without a population center or animals nearby. There are heavily trafficked areas such as the staging area on Denali or the foot of the Khumbu Icefall, where I advise caution. Do not wait for thirst to signal the need to drink as this mechanism may not work well up high.

EFFECTS OF ALTITUDE ILLNESS

1. *I went on a trek to altitude in Nepal and wasn't feeling well. I don't recall the details, but a helicopter was called and I was evacuated. When I arrived in Kathmandu, I felt perfectly fine. I should not be liable to pay the rescue bill, since I really wasn't sick there. Isn't it up to the agency and the trek leader to pay for it?*

You should gratefully pay for being alive. Such common stories indicate the person had a form of altitude illness requiring descent that was promptly carried out resulting in a rapid response and a survivor. The leader should be thanked for exercising conservative judgment, which is prudent at altitude. There are too many situations where people waited too long, and bodies were evacuated. Ask your travel agent about rescue insurance before you leave.

2. I feel so awful, but it's getting dark. Can't I wait until morning to get down?

No. You are faced with a difficult decision. There are too many cases where a corpse was found in the morning to even suggest waiting.

3. I walked slowly from Lukla to Namche Bazaar, and I still got altitude illness. What should I do differently on my next trip to altitude?

It is not the speed of your walking, but the amount that you raise your sleeping altitude that counts. Sleep at Lukla the first night and at Jorsale the next before ascending to Namche. Do not carry a loaded pack the next time to limit exertion, as those who exercise at a more rapid rate may be more inclined to get AMS and HAPE.

4. Couldn't my breathing condition, cough, and fever be pneumonia at altitude? Shouldn't I wait to see if the antibiotics work?

No. It's best to treat all suspected cases of pneumonia at altitude as if they were HAPE and add an antibiotic to the regimen.

5. My Sherpa, Lhakpa, has rapid breathing, lethargy, and a cough. A high altitude native, he couldn't

have HAPE, could he?

Yes. He could have HAPE and will need to be treated as any other person with the same symptoms. Some lowlanders in Nepal call themselves Sherpa to get the business.

6. *Could my diarrhea be a symptom of altitude illness?*

Unlikely. Your water losses will be greater at altitude so hydrate more.

7. *I've had a cold that started before coming to altitude. Now the trip leader is concerned that I have HAPE. My symptoms seem the same. Could she be right?*

Yes. Others are often more capable than you to notice changes in signs of altitude.

8. *The trek leader listened to my lungs and told me she heard rales. Does this mean I have HAPE?*

No, rales (a particular sound, also called crackles, heard with a stethoscope on listening to the chest) are common at altitude and do not by themselves mean a person has HAPE. If crackles persist after several deep breaths, HAPE or pneumonia could be present. Look for other signs and symptoms.

9. *My companions tell me I have HAPE. I have descended a thousand feet to where I first began to feel the extreme shortness of breath. Now I feel a little better. Shouldn't I spend the night here and see how I feel in the morning?*

No. Such a scenario has proven fatal. When you have serious

symptoms of altitude illness, you should descend to below the altitude at which you first had any symptoms of altitude illness, even mild ones. You may not improve significantly before doing so.

10. *Everyone in my group, except me, got up several times last night to pee. I feel fine, what should I do? Drink more?*

Yes, you may well be dehydrated. Check for other symptoms of altitude illness as well, and act accordingly. Alert your companions that you are not urinating as much as they are. Ask that they watch you for possible signs of developing altitude illness.

11. *We were all short of breath ascending to the high point. Why all this fuss about me, continuing to be short of breath?*

It seems you didn't improve with rest, which is the key point. Those short of breath with activity should quickly get better with rest.

12. *I've climbed ten fourteen-thousanders in Colorado. That means I'll have no problems with altitude going to Everest Base Camp? Right?*

Unfortunately not. Response to altitude is variable from person to person, and for an individual from time to time. There are many Everest summiters who have since had serious symptoms of altitude illness at much lower elevations.

13.   I'm a doctor. I know what's going on, and I do not have altitude illness!

The mortality rate for doctors at high altitude is disproportionately greater.

14.   I notice that George in the next tent is short of breath all the time, even when resting. He eats very little at meals. He says he's fine. Should the rest of our group be concerned or take action?

Yes. It could be altitude illness denial. Go through the protocol and act accordingly, or get George down a few thousand feet and see if he improves.

15.   Sandra has been getting worse at altitude for the last few days. The leader says it's because she has the flu, is dehydrated, and hasn't been practicing her meditation exercises properly. What should we do?

Act on humanitarian grounds and get the leader to agree to have her descend without delay to see if she improves. If the leader refuses, consider going against the decision.

16.   Jeremiah died of presumed altitude causes in Dolpo. Shouldn't we do all we can to get the body back to his home?

No. Recognize how difficult it is to transport a corpse on carriers in many countries, impossible in some. Consider a proper traditional disposal of the remains according to the local customs. You will need to deal with local authorities and other survivors. Write down what happened, photograph everything, and save as many personal effects as possible.

WHO SHOULD GO TO ALTITUDE

1. I'm pregnant and want to go on a high altitude adventure. Is this wise?

We do not know about the effects of altitude on pregnancy to either the lowlander mother or the fetus. If there was a mishap in the pregnancy outcome that could be attributed to altitude, would you blame yourself? Then limit altitude exposure to 10,000 to 12,000 feet (3050 to 3660 meters) and ascend slowly, so you don't seriously compromise the amount of oxygen carried in the blood. A miscarriage in a remote area would be scary for most women.

2. Should I take my children to high altitude with me?

As more and more parents venture to altitude, children accompany them to altitudes of 18,000 feet (5500 meters) or so, without ill effect. A leisurely itinerary is important. Children aged three and seven have hiked to the top of Kala Pattar (18,450 feet, 5620 meters). A three-and-a-half year old was successfully treated for symptoms of lethargy in a hyperbaric bag. It is difficult to identify symptoms and signs of altitude illness in children. Altitude localities are cold and remote, making evacuation worrisome. Consider any questionable behavior at altitude to be altitude illness. Descend quickly and few problems should result.

3. Does it make sense to postpone the trip to altitude for a few years until we know more about the scourge of altitude illness?

We know what we need to know to prevent deaths from altitude illness.

4. *I have heart disease and a number of other medical problems, and I have had coronary bypass surgery. I take medicines for high blood pressure. My doctor tells me I shouldn't even think of going to Khumbu to see Mount Everest, though it has been a lifelong dream of mine. Should I listen to him?*

The answer depends on the benefits that you will gain from attaining your goal, weighed against the increased risk of being in a place where full-service emergency care is not minutes away. The chance of dying from heart disease does not appear to increase at altitude. If you decide to go, find a doctor who can advise you in modifying your blood pressure drugs at altitude if necessary. Travel with a group that includes altitude savants.

5. *Are individuals with migraine headaches more inclined to migraine headaches at altitude?*

Perhaps. Some people report an increased frequency, others greater severity with symptoms not seen lower down. Treat them as any other headache at altitude, checking for ataxia, rapid breathing, and so on. Don't ascend, and try pain medicine if there are no ominous findings.

FOR LEADERS OF EXPEDITIONS AND TRIPS TO ALTITUDE

What advice would you give to a leader who wants to minimize the risk of problems when taking a group of people to altitude?

■ Be especially familiar with the material in chapter 4, "Diagnosing Altitude Illness" on recognizing altitude illness in others.

- Be systematic and get a report from each person each day on how they are doing and feeling, and add comments from your own perspective. Write it down and include the sleeping altitude as well as the day's activity. You can refer to this later if you suspect that altitude illness is responsible for the problems a person is experiencing; it may prove helpful in reaching a conclusion. It's best to organize the information into a table before-hand with each person's name, their symptoms, your impressions, sleeping altitude, and activity.

- Be flexible in your itinerary to allow the slowest person to acclimatize.

- If you are heading up and weather and conditions are deteriorating, or your party is not acclimatizing well or can only marginally cope with the circumstances, reconsider the decision.

Glossary

acclimatization. The process of the body adapting to high altitude where there is less oxygen in the air to breathe.

acute mountain sickness (AMS). In the setting of a recent gain in altitude, the presence of headache and at least one of the following symptoms:

- gastrointestinal (poor or no appetite, nausea, or vomiting)
- fatigue or weakness
- dizziness or lightheadedness
- difficulty sleeping

altered mental status. A change in the level and functioning of the psyche (a person's intellectual functioning, including emotional, attitudinal, psychological, and personality aspects). For example, the person is not thinking clearly, and he may not be aware of external events or surroundings.

altitude illness. The totality of conditions associated with not feeling well at altitude.

ataxia. Altered balance and muscular coordination, resulting from the brain not working correctly. Check by performing the tandem walking test (see chapter 4, section III).

attitude illness. Denial of altitude illness because of concern for ego, self-image, and one's relationship with others in the group.

cyanosis. A bluer skin color than that of similarly complexioned companions reflecting the inability to transport oxygen adequately in the blood (in the daylight, compare the color of lips or fingernail beds).

disease. Literally a lack of ease, but understood as a disorder of physiological or psychological function in the biomedical model.

diuresis. An increase in urination.

extreme altitude. Elevations above 18,000 feet (5500 meters).

high altitude cerebral edema (HACE). In the setting of a recent gain in altitude, the presence of a change in mental status or ataxia or both in a person with AMS, or the presence of both mental status change and ataxia in a person without AMS.

high altitude edema. Swelling of the hands, face, or ankles at altitude.

high altitude pulmonary edema (HAPE). In the setting of a recent gain in altitude, the presence of at least two each of the following signs and symptoms:

signs:

- rales (crackles) or wheezing in at least one lung field
- central cyanosis
- rapid breathing
- rapid heartbeat

symptoms:

- shortness of breath at rest
- cough
- weakness or decreased exercise performance
- chest tightness or congesting

high altitude retinopathy. Changes in the retina of the eyes at altitude, in which there is bleeding and other pathology.

high altitude syncope. Fainting that occurs after eating and standing up in the first 24 hours after arrival to intermediate altitudes. The faint is followed by quick recovery. If it recurs, something else is going on.

illness. A state of feeling unwell.

intermediate altitude. Defined in this book as altitudes to 12,000 feet (3660 meters).

periodic breathing. During sleep, cyclical changes in the rate and depth of breathing from rapid and strong to weak and almost imperceptible.

pulse oximeter. A device applied to the fingertip that senses color to measure the percentage of red blood cells that are carrying oxygen (called the "finger test" by some).

sickness. A role bestowed upon an individual by a community or group characterized by some deficit in normal mental or physical function.

sign. What is externally observable in a sick person, usually taken to mean what a health practitioner sees, palpates, listens to, or measures.

symptoms. What a sick person feels or complains about.

syncope. Denoting a brief loss of consciousness; termed a faint.

syndrome. An association of symptoms and signs that occur together more often than would be expected by chance.

tandem walking test. A test for ataxia (see chapter 4, section III).

References

FOR NON-MEDICAL READERS

Bezruchka, S. 1999. *The Pocket Doctor: Your Ticket to Good Health while Traveling.* 3rd ed. Seattle: The Mountaineers Books.

Grissom, C. K. 1993. Medical therapy of high altitude illness. *American Alpine Journal* 35 (67): 118–23.

Hackett, P. H. 1980. *Mountain sickness: Prevention, recognition, and treatment.* 2nd ed. New York: American Alpine Club.

Houston, C. 2005. *Going higher: Oxygen, man, and mountains,* 5th ed. Seattle: The Mountaineers Books.

West, J. B. 2002. Unexplained severe fatigue and lassitude at high altitude. *High Altitude Medicine and Biology* 3 (2): 237–41.

FOR HEALTH PROFESSIONALS

Bezruchka, S. 1992. High altitude medicine. *Medical Clinics of North America* 76 (6): 1481–97.

Entin, P. L., and L. Coffin. 2004. Physiological basis for recommendations regarding exercise during pregnancy at high altitude. *High Altitude Medicine and Biology* 5 (3): 321–34.

Hornbein, T., and R. B. Schoene, eds. 2001. High altitude: An exploration of human adaptation. *Lung Biology in Health and Disease Vol. 161.* New York: Marcel Dekker.

Hultgren, H. 1997. *High altitude medicine.* Stanford: Hultgren Publications.

Lee, A. G., R. Anderson, R. H. Kardon, M. Wall. 2004. Presumed "sulfa allergy" in patients with intracranial hypertension treated with acetazolamide or furosemide: cross-reactivity, myth or reality? *American Journal of Ophthalmology* 138 (1): 114–18.

Levine, B. D. 2002. Intermittent hypoxic training: Fact and fancy. *High Altitude Medicine and Biology* 3 (2): 177–93.

Levine, B. D., J. H. Zuckerman, and C. R. diFilippi. 1997. Effect of high-altitude exposure in the elderly: the Tenth Mountain Division study. *Circulation* 96 (4): 1224–32.

Mader, T. H., and G. Tabin. 2003. Going to high altitude with preexisting ocular conditions. *High Altitude Medicine and Biology* 4 (4): 419–30.

Pollard, A. J., S. Niermeyer, et al. 2001. Children at high altitude: an international consensus statement by an ad hoc committee of the International Society for

Mountain Medicine, March 12, 2001. *High Altitude Medicine and Biology* 2 (3): 389–403.

Pollard, A. J., and D. R. Murdoch. 2003. *The high altitude medicine handbook.* Oxford: Radcliffe Medical Press.

Shlim, D. R., and J. Gallie. 1992. The causes of death among trekkers in Nepal. *International Journal of Sports Medicine* 13 (Supp 1): S74–S76.

Ward, M. P., J. S. Milledge, and J. B. West. 2000. *High altitude medicine and physiology.* New York: Oxford University Press.

Index

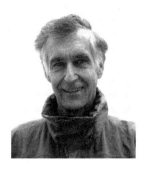

About the Author

Stephen Bezruchka has lived at altitude and has ascended to extreme altitudes. He has climbed in Canada, the United States, China, Pakistan, and Nepal. A board-certified emergency physician, he has also worked in the fields of travel medicine and international health. In Nepal he set up a community health project in a remote area, conducted a clinical teaching program for Nepali doctors in a rural district hospital, and consulted on health projects. He is the author of *The Pocket Doctor: Your Ticket to Good Health While Traveling, Trekking in Nepal: A Traveler's Guide*, and *Nepali for Trekkers,* all available from The Mountaineers Books. He received degrees from the University of Toronto as well as from Harvard, Stanford, and Johns Hopkins Universities. Currently he is on the faculty of the Department of Health Services at the University of Washington, where he's working on drawing attention to the poor health status of the United

States in comparison to other rich countries, and the reasons therefore (see *depts.washington.edu/eqhlth*). He is a member of the American Alpine Club, the Alpine Club of Canada, the International Society for Mountain Medicine, and the Wilderness Medical Society. And he has qualified to join the Supine Alpine Club. The entry requirements for men are to have suffered from AML (Acute Mountain Lassitude), CPF (Congestive Prostate Failure), TT (Terminal Torpor), and HAFE.

Founded in 1906, The Mountaineers is a Seattle-based non-profit outdoor activity and conservation club with 15,000 members, whose mission is "to explore, study, preserve, and enjoy the natural beauty of the outdoors . . . ." The club sponsors many classes and year-round outdoor activities in the Pacific Northwest, and supports environmental causes by sponsoring legislation and presenting educational programs. The Mountaineers Books supports the club's mission by publishing travel and natural history guides, instructional texts, and works on conservation and history. For information, call or write The Mountaineers, Club Headquarters, 300 Third Avenue West, Seattle, Washington, 98119; (206) 284-6310.

Send or call for our catalog of more than 500 outdoor titles:

The Mountaineers Books
1001 SW Klickitat Way, Suite 201
Seattle, WA 98134
800-553-4453
mbooks@mountaineersbooks.org
www.mountaineersbooks.org

The Mountaineers Books is proud to be a corporate sponsor of The Leave No Trace Center for Outdoor Ethics, whose mission is to promote and inspire responsible outdoor recreation through education, research, and partnerships. The Leave No Trace program is focused specifically on human-powered (nonmotorized) recreation.

Leave No Trace strives to educate visitors about the nature of their recreational impacts, as well as offer techniques to prevent and minimize such impacts. Leave No Trace is best understood as an educational and ethical program, not as a set of rules and regulations.

For more information, visit *www.LNT.org,* or call 800-332-4100.

MORE TITLES YOU MIGHT ENJOY FROM THE MOUNTAINEERS BOOKS

Going Higher: Oxygen, Man, and Mountains, 5th Edition, *Charles Houston, M.D., David Harris, Ph.D., Ellen Zeman, Ph.D.* How the body responds to high altitude—this classic study, now in its fifth edition, is the most definitive book on the topic.

Hypothermia, Frostbite and Other Cold Injuries: Prevention Recognition, Prehospital Treatment, *James Wilkerson, M.D.* Symptoms, solutions, and prevention described by experts.

Medicine for Mountaineering & Other Wilderness Activities, 4th Edition
James Wilkerson, M.D.
A classic since 1967, this book starts where most first-aid manuals stop.

Glacier Travel & Crevasse Rescue, 2nd Edition, *Andy Selters*
Packed with information by a trainer for the American Alpine Institute.
A must-read before stepping onto a glacier.

Mountain Weather: Backcountry Forecasting and Weather Safety for Hikers, Campers, Climbers, Skiers, Snowboarders, *Jeff Renner*
Learn to read mountain weather and you'll stay safer and enjoy your time there more.

Mountaineering First Aid: A Guide to Accident Response and First Aid Care, 5th Edition,
Jan Carline, Ph.D., Steven MacDonald, M.P.H., Ph.D., and Martha Lentz, R.N., Ph.D.
Expert first-aid instruction used extensively by the American Red Cross.
